Down the Plughole

Down the Plughole

An irreverent history of the bath

Steve Dobell

First published in Great Britain in 1996 by
PAVILION BOOKS LIMITED
26 Upper Ground, London SE1 9PD

Text design by Cole design unit

A CIP catalogue record for this book is
available from the British Library

ISBN 1 85793 981 6

Typeset in 9½/11pt Stempel Garamond by
Dorchester Typesetting Group Limited
Printed and bound in Great Britain by
BPC Consumer Books

2 4 6 8 10 9 7 5 3 1

This book may be ordered by post direct from
the publisher.
Please contact the Marketing Department.
But try your bookshop first.

Contents

Introduction
or Running In

You can't beat a good hot bath. It is one of life's great sensual pleasures and one of its most democratic luxuries. You do not, after all, need asses' milk, like the Emperor Nero's wife Poppaea and, supposedly, Cleopatra, to enjoy a sense of total relaxation and pampered wellbeing. It is also a sensible way of keeping the body clean. Few nowadays would dispute this, nor would many ancient races, from Mexicans to Minoans, for whom it was obvious. Yet this simple fact has eluded entire civilizations, just as in our own times the non-Francophone world has largely missed the point about the bidet.

One result of this intermittent balneological myopia is that the history of baths and bathing makes odd reading. For anyone who believes in the inevitability of progress, and in the perfectibility of the human race and all its works, it tends to throw a spanner in them, for the story is not so much linear as circular. Whereas the history of aviation, for example, begins with an optimist standing on a hill flapping ludicrously inadequate wings, continues with huge constructions of balsa wood and canvas, held together with string, Sellotape and chewing gum, which collapse in a heap, and only after much labour and heroism culminates in the glory of Concorde and the Stealth bomber, the history of the bath begins, as it were, with Concorde and then goes straight back to Alcock and Brown. It has taken over 1,500 years to rectify the situation. What is more, as we shall see, although the technology of bathing may now at last be more advanced then ever, in many ways this new zenith is not as remarkable as the old one. For in Ancient Greece and Rome baths, and especially public baths, had a significance in daily life that they have never been accorded since.

It is partly just a matter of scale. There is a world of difference, after all, between a modern public swimming pool or a health club – or even the Empire Pool, Wembley – and baths built on such a grand scale that, centuries after the sack of Rome, their ruins could grip the imagination of a Shelley. When New York and London are eventually laid low, it seems unlikely that the remains of their bathing establishments will long delay the lyric poets of the thirty-third century.

Much more significant, however, is the matter of attitude. A telling illustration is provided by a recently published book on British writers and their houses. Had the book been about Roman writers, one could be sure that its contributors would have dwelt admiringly on the bathing facilities which helped support each writer's health and morale. Behind each great writer they would have found a great bath, or more likely the minimum trinity of caldarium, tepidarium and frigidarium. No such inspiration for the British scribes, however. We may leave aside the fact that when Virginia and Leonard Woolf arrived at Monk's House, as when George Bernard Shaw came to Shaw's Corner and T. E. Lawrence to Clouds Hill, there was no water supply – though this in itself speaks volumes. More to the point, in the descriptions of the remaining 50-odd houses the *only references* to baths or bathing are to the effect that Thomas Carlyle would shower himself with cold water in the back kitchen, Vanessa Bell made do with a basin of water (frozen in winter), and Thomas Hardy had lived for many years at Max Gate – which was built to his own design – when his second wife Florence 'introduced a bathroom'. Indeed we are as likely to read about billiard tables as baths. We are left in no doubt that even if creature comforts are provided for, such provision is not thought worthy of comment.

Nowadays all that has changed, and greater luxury and sophistication are available in our bathrooms than even the

Romans knew – for those who are interested. This is the crux of the matter. For unlike the loo, whose history has been one of steady development from smelly garderobe to the almost silent flush, the bathtub has changed little in its essentials since Minoan times. It is basically a container, which is either full or empty, and its history has less to do with its contours or accessories than with people's fluctuating attitudes to filling it. In writing about bathing habits, moreover, it is hardly ever possible to be categorical. A king, for example, may have had a luxurious bath at a time when none of his subjects even considered bathing. On the other hand, the fact that he installed one in his palace doesn't mean that his successor ever used it. Indeed, there is often no way of knowing whether he ever used it himself. Having a bath is one thing; taking a bath is another. These are deep waters.

The one certainty about the bath is that we need it. It is time to get in.

1
Improving Baths

In our cultural humility we in western Europe tend to think that we owe almost every attribute of our civilization to the Ancient Greeks – even if in some cases the Chinese had them first. It does seem to be more or less true that we ourselves invented nothing of significance before cricket and the steam engine, and that most of the things we hold dear – from grammar and democracy to snakes-and-ladders – were indeed supplied to us (via the Romans or even the French) by the people at the shallow end of the Mediterranean. It is a pleasant novelty, therefore, to be able to say that while the Greeks were among the early leading players in the steamy drama that is the history of the bath, they did not in fact turn on the tap.

The Minoans of Crete and the Hittites of Anatolia were definitely in there first. The earliest known bathtub dates from about 1700BC and is to be found at the palace of King Minos at Knossos – where Theseus confronted the Minotaur – in a superbly ornate bathroom in the Queen's apartments. The whole palace had terracotta plumbing, and although the Queen's bath was essentially just a simple ceramic container, similar in shape to the modern bath, and hot water, if any, would have had to be carried to the bath from the cauldron, it was sumptuously decorated inside and out. In any case, who needs taps or plughole when you have bevies of servants on hand to top you up? Not that the plughole was beyond the Minoan imagination. At a tavern nearby other baths of the same period have been found which were indeed plumbed in for the convenience of do-it-yourself bathers.

Hot on the heels of the Minoans – in the history of bathing, that is – came the Hittites. Uriah and Bathsheba

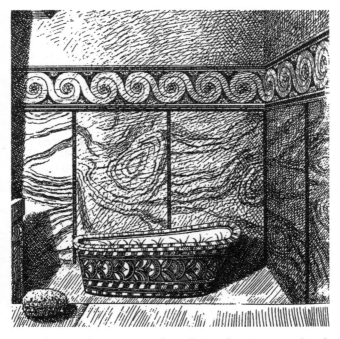

A royal receptacle at Knossos, the earliest and most spectacular of terracotta bathtubs.

(see page 89), now the most famous of their race, were not alone in appreciating the merits of bathing. In the late Bronze Age, when the Hittite Empire was among the most powerful in the Middle East, it appears that many of their more luxurious homes had bathrooms. In the town of Alaca, in the Hatti region of Anatolia (now central Turkey), square-shaped terracotta bathtubs dating from about 1500BC have been found, some so small that they must have been for children. Others had built-in seats, anticipating the sit-up bath favoured to this day by the

French. The Hittites, like the Minoans, also had terracotta drains consisting of tapering sections of pipe which fitted one inside the other.

The Ancient Greeks were undoubtedly the first to make baths a public institution as well as a private luxury and, as one might expect, to develop a philosophy of bathing. (One of them, as we shall see, even made use of the bath to achieve a scientific breakthrough.) They too used terracotta baths, and at the late Hellenic palace of Tiryns archaeologists found a remarkable bathroom containing several such baths. The floor of the room consisted of a single block of limestone, weighing twenty tons, with a raised edge and a gentle slope towards one corner, from which the water drained. As early as 500BC the palace of Vouni, in Cyprus, was equipped with a number of bathrooms where, as well as latrines, there were both hot and cold baths. We also know from contemporary accounts that hot water was provided in public baths at Sybaris, another Greek possession on the coast of southern Italy, until its destruction in 510BC. The Sybarites' lifestyle was one of fabled luxury, and for them to have missed out on the hot bath would have been an uncharacteristic oversight.

Legend has it that Greeks were enjoying hot baths well before this time. According to Homer, during the siege of Troy many centuries earlier the Trojan hero Hector, returning home after a hard day's fighting against Agamemnon's army, would slip into a hot bath before dinner. After that long campaign Ulysses is described having a well-deserved bath on his protracted voyage back to Ithaca, while Agamemnon himself, on his return to Sparta – feeling no doubt that he too had earned a good long soak – stepped into the bath that was to prove fatal. His wife Clytemnestra, herself unfaithful, was so incensed by reports of his dalliance with Cassandra at Troy that she hacked him to death with an axe.

Generally the Greeks favoured cold baths, and bathing

was regarded as a healthy adjunct to vigorous exercise. Indeed bathing facilities normally formed part of an all-round educational establishment known as a gymnasium. This would include an exercise ground called a palestra, where they engaged in wrestling and other gymnastic pursuits, and a semi-circular exedra, for the mental and verbal wrestling of debates and philosophical discussions. Although the baths, usually located between the two, consisted at first of little more than cold showers and foot-baths hollowed out along a rudimentary marble trough, one presumably emerged from the gymnasium feeling physically, intellectually and morally refreshed. As time went on, plunge baths were provided, and soon the gymnasium began to be built on a much larger scale, inside huge vaulted halls which anticipated the Roman thermae.

The object of the exercise, however, was still exercise and regeneration, not hedonism. Although hot baths gradually became more popular, the Greeks would dutifully take their invigorating cold bath first. At Oenidae, in Acarnia, as early as the second century BC, the arrangement that would become the norm for the Romans was already established: a frigidarium, with a small square plunge pool of cold water; a tepidarium, a big round room with eight individual basins sunk into the floor; and a caldarium, a smaller room, also round, with numerous basins of steaming hot water. Hot water was produced, according to Herodotus, by means of red-hot irons or heated stones.

Gradually the Greeks had to admit that the pleasure principle could no longer be overlooked. A warm bath was not just good for tired muscles – it was awfully nice. At Olympia in about 100BC they even began to heat the basement and the walls, which meant that in cold weather, when there was little comfort to be had at home, the public baths provided a warm haven. Although even in Athens the public baths were never built on anything like the scale of the Roman thermae, they were luxurious and welcoming. The baths themselves were sometimes made of glass, but usually of marble or bronze, which was especially good for retaining heat.

This was becoming a congenial place to linger. As a result, while the richer citizens would certainly have their own baths, often even with hot water, the public baths remained a popular social institution for anyone who could afford to pay. Some would come several times a day, and when using the hot baths you would enjoy the services of a scantily clad male attendant, who would pour on the water and afterwards anoint your body with aromatic oils. The public baths were especially popular with women. Order and proportion prevailed, even so, and there was strict segregation of the sexes – a detail which the Romans, when borrowing the custom, often saw fit to overlook.

For one Greek bather, Archimedes, a discovery made in the bath provided not only instant satisfaction but a place in scientific history. Archimedes was a philosopher who lived at Syracuse, in Sicily, in the third century BC, when it was a province of Greece. One day he had been wrestling with a thorny problem and getting nowhere, so he went to the baths, as freelancers do, just to get away from it all. However, the problem was still revolving in his mind, and just as he was getting into his warm bath for a final soak the answer came to him in a flash.

He had been employed to find out whether a consignment of gold, supplied for the creation of a crown for King Hiero, was in fact pure gold, or had been adulterated. He would be able to tell by the weight, of course, but only if he knew the gold's volume, or mass – which he didn't. As he lowered himself into the bath, and the water level rose, it suddenly came to him: the volume of the water displaced by his body (or any body) must be equal to that of the body. If the gold were to be totally immersed in water inside a regular-shaped container such as a cylinder, the volume could be measured. 'By Jove!' he cried, and leaped out of the bath. Forgetting about such banal details as getting dressed or tipping the attendant, he then ran home to put his Displacement Theory to the test, shouting '*Eureka*!' – meaning 'I've cracked it!' – by way of explanation to bemused passers-by. His flight was no doubt accompanied by ribald comments such as 'ἄφρων ποραπαιςι'[1] and 'ἐκεῖδς ἐφυγε',[2] but history has been kinder, casting Archimedes in the role of the original dotty professor.

---

1. 'It's a loony!'
2. 'She went that way!'

2
Marble Halls

Anything the Greeks could do, the Romans could do better. That, at least, was the impression they strove to create. In fact the Romans had, for all their vast Empire, a cultural inferiority complex *vis-à-vis* the Greeks, and they tried to compensate by building on an ostentatiously grand scale. The well-known saying, 'Ἑνδεκσ γαρ δυναται Πολυφημους Μῶνος Οδυδδευς'[1] meant little to the Romans. Compared with the Greek baths, the Romans' were bigger and better too, but their bathing was no longer a serene Arcadian idyll. Nor was it any longer just one part of the gymnasium experience, sandwiched between exercise and philosophical discussion. Education gradually took second place to simple enjoyment, and, increasingly, to sensuality and vanity. They did, however, know how to enjoy themselves, and they took the art of hedonistic bathing to a scale and a sophistication never seen before or since.

The basic components of the early Roman baths, public and private alike, were broadly similar to those of the Greeks, but the emphasis had changed. The stadium in which they were situated would still include a palestra for athletics, and often a theatre and a library, but the baths themselves were now pre-eminent.

They consisted of a series of rooms, each at a different temperature and serving a specific purpose. The principle was that after a work-out in the palestra one would enter one of the apodyteria, or dressing-rooms, and strip for action, then rest for a while in the moderate heat of the tepidarium, which opened the pores. Next one moved to the caldarium, where the temperature was higher, and took a hot bath, before entering the seriously hot air (over 200°F) of the sudatorium or laconicum (named after the Lace-daemonians, who apparently invented hot-air bathing). Now it was time to be anointed with oils and unguents, massaged and scraped clean with a curved metal tool known as a strigil. After that it must have been a pleasant relief to plunge into the big cold pool of the frigidarium. This was where most of the socializing went on.

Not that the baths were used purely for bathing and socializing. Most people, it is true, did just that; the baths opened at midday, and they would turn up early in the afternoon at the end of the day's work. Others took their work with them, and floating desks enabled them to get on with paperwork or hold meetings. They were probably about as popular as those who take their mobile phones into places of entertainment today.

The sequence of rooms was replicated on a smaller scale at bathing establishments in towns and villas, perhaps without the apodyterium and laconicum. One Roman patrician who had her own laconicum was St Cecilia, one of the early Christian martyrs. The story goes that during one of the persecutions Cecilia steadfastly refused to renounce her faith and was sentenced to be roasted alive in her own bathroom. In spite of prodigious heat she apparently survived for three days before eventually being beheaded by her exhausted executioners.

The water for the baths was originally heated by braziers. In the first century BC, however, the Romans had made their great breakthrough with the invention of an under-floor heating system called a hypocaust. This was a hollow space beneath the floor, which rested on pillars of brick. It was heated, together with the water tank, by a furnace, or in a large establishment by several. Later the walls, too, were built hollow and heated with hot air carried in square earthenware pipes. This highly effective all-round heating system distributed heat evenly throughout the room. Its capacity for heating a building of any size, together with the engineers' triumphant spanning of ever wider spaces with domes and arches, made possible the giant thermae. For the next few centuries, these, with their increasing size and splendour, represented state-of-the-art Roman technology.

At the time of Augustus (27BC–AD14), the thermae, like everything in Roman life, were a model of order and decorum. The rules governing bathing in public were as strict as in Greece, in fact more so. For fear of immorality, not only were the sexes segregated, which ruled out the opportunity for such a crime; at one time it was even decreed that the attendants in the women's baths had to be eunuchs, which, as far as heterosexual hanky-panky went, removed means and motive as well.

Subsequently, especially with the popularity of the superb large-scale thermae, of which the first were built by Nero, Titus and Domitian in the first century AD, standards began to slip. So dramatic was this moral decadence that in the third century the Emperor Gallienus not only allowed bathing to be mixed as well as completely nude, but regularly joined in. In fact there was nothing unusual about an emperor frolicking with his subjects; some found it so diverting that their meals would be served in the water; others had foibles that were rather less savoury. Contemporary writers of several periods hinted obliquely at goings-on so depraved and revolting that . . . well, they could only be hinted at obliquely. Ours not to speculate about such matters, but since we know that Caligula's horse was made a senator and could thus walk the corridors of power, it is reasonable to assume that he was also free to strut his stuff at the baths.

Not that the history of bathing in Rome was one of continuous moral decline. Policy would change according to the tastes and mood of whoever ruled, so that periods of more or less uncontrolled promiscuity would alternate with more disciplined regimes. Moreover, the baths were

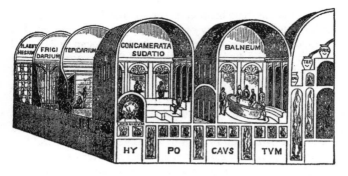

A Roman diagram of a bath-house, with the hypocaust clearly shown.

so extensive that, whatever the prevailing moral climate, it was normally possible, for those who wished, to find more conservative bathing facilities without the distractions of nudity or the opposite sex. Failing that, the wealthy could always fall back on their private baths at home, but life in the capital, in contrast to that in the country or in distant outposts of the Empire, was never really complete without a visit to the public baths once, if not several times a day.

If the Romans were bent on outdoing the Greeks, they were also very competitive among themselves. The increasingly vast and magnificent thermae symbolized each emperor's determination to go one better than his predecessor. The earliest large-scale thermae of which ruins survive are the Baths of Titus, built on the site of the palace of Nero, overlooking the Colosseum, during the short reign of the popular and moderate Emperor Titus. They were begun in AD79, the year that saw the destruction of Pompeii and Herculaneum.

Much more imposing are the ruins of the Baths of Caracalla. The Emperor Caracalla was among the most brutal and barbaric of all the emperors (at the age of 23 he murdered his half-brother Geta so that he could be sole ruler), but in the history of bathing he has to be regarded as something of a hero. The baths which he began in 212, and which were finished off by Alexander Severus about twenty years later, were far bigger than anything the world had ever seen, with an area roughly six times that of St Paul's Cathedral. Built at the foot of the Aventine Hill, and supplied with water by the Antonine Aqueduct, this enormous edifice, with its towering domes, arches and vaulting, could accommodate 1,600 bathers in its numerous rooms and had marble seating for 2,000 spectators. The interior was quite spectacular: built of granite and green marble, it had vast windows of glass to let in light, walls covered in mosaics, and water flowing into the basins from silver spouts. Patricians and plebeians alike must have felt like princes.

The grandeur of the baths can be gauged from the reactions of those who saw the ruins in their more complete state. For the poet Percy Bysshe Shelley, who was living in Rome in the spring of 1819, the majestic ruins provided an inspirational setting for the composition of his great lyric drama *Prometheus Unbound*. He wrote in the Preface:

This Poem was chiefly written upon the mountainous ruins of the Baths of Caracalla, among the flowery glades, and thickets of odiferous blossoming trees, which are extended in ever winding labyrinths upon its immense platforms and dizzy arches suspended in the air. The bright blue sky of Rome, and the effect of the vigorous awakening spring in that divinest climate, and the new life with which it drenches the spirits even to intoxication, were the inspiration of this drama.

The greatest, or most extensive thermae, however, were yet to come. By the fourth century AD the Empire was well into its decline, but there was still sufficient wealth for the erection of monuments of prodigious scale. Between 302 and 309 the Emperor Diocletian, the notorious persecutor of the Christians, used more than ten thousand of them as slave labour in the construction of a massive complex of baths on the Quirinal Hill. Nearly a mile in circumference, they are said to have had room for twice as many customers as the Baths of Caracalla. What the noise levels must have been like in these establishments, with all the laughing and shouting – quite apart from their moral tone – scarcely bears thinking about. A visiting Greek, accustomed to the refined ambience of the gymnasium, would have suffered thunderous culture shock and, in his letter home, might well have quoted Theocritus – 'ὄχλος ἄθρως. ὤθεῦνθ ὤεπερ ὕες.'[2]

In Renaissance times, when the Baths of Diocletian also lay abandoned, a Sicilian priest claimed to have seen the Virgin Mary, accompanied by a group of angels, wandering among the ruins. Presumably they cannot have had towels under their arms, for the vision was interpreted as a sign, not that she thought it was time for the baths to be restored, but rather that it was a good place for a church. Perhaps Mary felt this was the best way of expunging the site's unseemly anti-Christian past. Michelangelo concurred, and proceeded to convert one of the main halls, probably the tepidarium, into the church of Santa Maria degli Angeli. His creation was heavily altered, unfortunately, in the eighteenth century.

In about 320, under Constantine, there were no fewer than eleven thermae and 856 private baths, catering to a population of about one-and-a-half million, while eleven great aqueducts were bringing into the city about one-and-a-half thousand million litres of water every day. The Baths of Constantine, a monument to one of the most remarkable of all Romans, were the last of the great thermae to be built, for, having made this contribution to epic-scale bathing, the Emperor would later proceed to hole it, as it were, below the waterline. Christianity was spreading rapidly through the Empire when Constantine began his reign, and it was under his auspices that it was recognized as the religion of the Empire. Constantine was himself baptized at the age of 65. History does not relate whether the ceremony took place in the baths he built – and if so at what temperature – or elsewhere, but we do know that it involved his total immersion in a state of complete nudity. This was a man who believed in doing things properly.

His other momentous action was to build up, and in 330 transfer power to, the Empire's second capital at Byzantium, which became known as the City of Constantine, later Constantinople, and would continue to be the capital of the Empire for many centuries. Less important historically, but a landmark in our story, was that following his conversion Constantine issued an edict forbidding mixed bathing. Hadrian and others had done this before him, but this time the prohibition stuck. This can be seen as one of the first baleful effects of Christianity on bathing history, and if it seemed at the time like the end of an era, that was not so very far from the truth. In the following century the Barbarians arrived in the Campagna and destroyed the aqueducts, the great lifelines which supplied Rome with its precious water, and long before the city fell, its bathing days were over. Perhaps the shock of this blow to Roman morale may have hastened what really was the end.

---

1. 'Size isn't everything.'
2. 'My dear, the noise – and the *people*!'

3
Imperial Bathers

The Romans took their bathing habits with them wherever their Empire spread, rather as the British, many centuries later, would export their cricket and other games to all corners of the globe. Surprisingly, whereas Britain's curious games often put down deep and permanent roots, the Romans never instilled their eminently sensible bathing ethic nearly as effectively. This may be due to the fact that whereas the British would have needed natives to make up the numbers for their games, whose rules were also quite easily grasped, the Romans were not for the most part eager to share their bathing facilities with Gauls, Africans and Ancient Britons, who may in turn have been daunted by the technology of the hypocaust.

For the Romans, of course, the bath was much more than a recreation or a mod con – it was a *sine qua non*. At a practical level, those in command were well aware that a refreshed, relaxed Roman soldier was always going to be more effective than an itchy, aching one. It was also an important morale-booster, and the further north the Romans ventured, into chilly, alien regions, the more welcoming and comforting their baths must have seemed. Nowhere more so than in Britain, arguably the least hospitable of all the conquered lands. The taming of Gaul had been arduous enough, but at least it was on the same landmass as Rome.

When the invasion of Britain began in AD43, nearly a century after Caesar's expeditions there, the invaders were entering virtually unknown territory. Setting out across the grey Channel, their thoughts must have turned nostalgically homewards: to the sun-drenched hills, balmy evenings by the Tiber, languid afternoons relaxing at the baths. Pressing on stoically, they advanced across the country, heroically replicating as far as possible the Roman way of life, or at least its bare necessities. Every fort and garrison was equipped with its bath-house, and as towns and cities grew up, bathing facilities were provided for civilians too. Remains of Roman bath-houses have been found in London, York, Bath, Wroxeter, Lincoln, Silchester and many other towns. In rural areas, no villa was complete without its suite of bathing rooms. It appears that in the South Wales gold mines there may even have been baths at the pit-head.

One can only guess what the Ancient Britons made of it all. They had doubtless been happy enough in their own way, living in their cosy mud huts, hunting for food, worshipping fire, water and other sensible things, sitting around the fire of an evening singing songs of battle. As far as personal hygiene was concerned, they held to the conviction that an occasional bit of grooming with twigs or animal bones was perfectly satisfactory. Then came these horribly well-organized foreigners, clearing the trees away, laying out towns, erecting buildings of unnecessary size and, most extraordinary of all, channelling precious water away from the streams, heating it, filling vast containers with it, and then sitting in it or worse. In some places in the south of the country the natives were even expected to follow suit. For many that was going too far.

Time and again, just when the more malleable southern Britons seemed to have been subdued and partly civilized, another rebellion would break out. Gradually, however, these outbreaks of insubordination became fewer, and the Romans were able to bring stability to much of the country and begin the long process of convincing the Briton of the value of the bath. It was only in the mountainous regions to the north and west that the inexorable advance of the legions was proving after all to be exorable.

Such was still the situation in AD120 when the Emperor

Hadrian visited this northern outpost of Empire. Hadrian was a thinker and a realist, whose travels around the Empire had already persuaded him that the time had come for a change of policy. He saw no reason to continue to extend its frontiers through conquest of intractable tribes. Far better, he thought, to consolidate what they already had, sealing the borders where necessary with impregnable defences, so that those within could live in harmony, bathe as often as possible and pay taxes.

On arrival in Britain, Hadrian could not only see which way the wind was blowing, he could smell it. Not to put too fine a point on it, he was appalled by the stench, especially from the north, and immediately put olfactory reform high on his list of priorities. Briefings from local commanders and hygienists convinced him that there was little to be done in the short term about the sanitary habits of the Picts, and nothing at all about the Scots, but he was determined to clear the air. Drastic defensive measures were called for, if only to maintain standards in the south. The solution was a continuous chain of fortified bathhouses stretching right across the country from coast to coast and linked by a wall. This sanitary curtain (still in existence, but sadly neglected) came to be known as Hadrian's Wall, and foolhardy was the legionary who ventured beyond it.

Some years later, such was the enthusiasm with which the baths were being patronized, Hadrian felt it necessary to issue an edict forbidding mixed bathing anywhere in the Empire – an intrusion that must have been about as welcome as some of the pronouncements issuing from Brussels in the late twentieth century. Nowhere would the effects of this edict have been felt more keenly than in Bath. With its hot sulphur spring and its convenient position on the main Fosse Way between Exeter and Lincoln, Bath had quickly developed in the first century AD into one of the major bathing centres of Europe. The Romans named the town Aquae Sulis, which means Waters of Sul, after the ancient goddess of the spring, whom they not only adopted but honoured by the erection of the temple of Sul-Minerva. It was a walled town, but seems to have been neither an important garrison nor an administrative centre. Rather it was purely a centre for health, rest and recreation, to which soldiers and civilians came from all over Britain and northern Gaul, many of them probably suffering from rheumatism brought on by the cold, damp climate. They would swim in the Great Bath, whose diving platform can still be seen, soak in the smaller Circular Bath, or sweat it out in the caldarium.

Nor were the baths used only by the Romans. While Agricola was ruler of Britain in AD78–84, Aquae Sulis had played an important role in his policy of Romanization, aimed at softening up and sanitizing the unruly Britons, or at least their leaders. The historian Tacitus describes his cunning plan:

In order that a race of rude and primitive men, versed in the arts of war, might be rendered peaceful and tranquil through the delights of luxury, he privately encouraged and officially helped them to build temples, market-places, and houses, praising the eager and admonishing the slothful. And so imitation became a matter of compulsion. For now, indeed, he instructed the sons of chieftains in the liberal arts and confronted British native wit with Gallic learning, so that only those that were unfamiliar with the Roman tongue were regarded as lacking in eloquence. Then they were made to adopt our style of dressing and the toga became common. Little by little they were lured to the blandishments of vice, to porticoes and baths, and to luxurious feasts. In this way an unsophisticated people learnt to mistake the path of servitude for the highroad to culture.

While Buxton played a similar R & R role for troops in the north, albeit without the benefit of a hot spring, Bath was undoubtedly the Romans' favourite place in Britain. It is curious to think that the very feature which made it so popular with the Romans, namely its water, also led to its becoming the favourite stamping ground of polite society in the England of Smollett and Jane Austen.

Although unrivalled in Britain, Aquae Sulis was by no means unique in Roman Europe. The Romans were adept at sniffing out hot springs, and bathing resorts sprang up wherever they found them. Many European towns which became famous spas in the eighteenth and nineteenth centuries were originally Roman bathing centres. Among them were Baden-Baden (Aquae Aureliae) and Wiesbaden (Aquae Mattiacum) in Germany, Baden (Aquae Helvetiae) near Zurich in Switzerland, and Aix-les-Bains (Aquae Allobrogum) and Aix-en-Provence (Aquae Sextiae) in France, all of which had warm or hot springs. One place which did not was Arles, but in the fourth century it had the biggest bathing establishment in Provence. Water was brought in by a 47-mile aqueduct, was supplied to the public baths and fountains, was used to flush the public urinals (built of white marble), and was also metred into private houses. In Paris (Lutetia Parisiorum) a very substantial bathing establishment was built early in the third century by the guild of Gallo-Roman boatmen; by the end of the century it had been destroyed by the Barbarians; its remains can still be seen beneath the Hôtel de Cluny, a former bishop's residence which was built on the site, just off the Boulevard St-Michel.

While in cities it was normal to use the public facilities, in rural areas bathing was very much a private luxury. The fourth-century writer Ausonius, who lived in Trier, provides a breathless description of palatial villas perched on rocky sites overlooking the Moselle. It is interesting to know that the gaunt medieval castles which seem to have dominated the region since time immemorial were in fact preceded by a kind of Roman Millionaires' Row, for he goes on:

*What need to make mention of their courts set beside
verdant meadows, of their trim roofs resting upon countless
pillars? What of their baths, contrived low down on the
verge of the bank, which smoke when Vulcan, drawn by
the glowing flue, pants forth his flames and whirls them up
through the channelled walls, rolling in masses the
imprisoned smoke before the scorching blast! I myself have
seen some, exhausted by the intense heat of the baths, scorn
the pools and cold plunge-baths, preferring to enjoy running
water, and, straightway refreshed by the river, buffet the
cool stream, threshing it with their stroke.*

When the Romans finally pulled back from their
provinces, it appears that virtually everything they left
behind was either destroyed or left to crumble. The fate of
Roman London, for example, remains a mystery, but is
likely to have been violent and sudden. Whatever happened, it seems that the art of heating, piping and enjoying
water was completely lost. Once the Romans had gone,
and the natives had reverted to smearing their bodies with
goose grease, the best that could be said about the sanitation of the British and the Saxons was that it would have
been a good idea.

4
Next to Godliness

In Dark Age Britain, nowhere was the darkness blacker than in the bathroom. This was largely because that room now ceased to exist, except spasmodically in palaces and so forth, for almost 1,500 years. When the Romans left Britain in 410, recalled to defend their capital against the Goths and Vandals, they might just as well have taken their baths with them, for they were quickly destroyed and forgotten. The Christianized Britons, who might have been expected to keep the water running, ran off themselves, driven west into Cornwall and Wales by the Anglo-Saxon invaders, who cared nothing for the natives' religion nor the Romans' baths.

Even if Britain had then remained Christian, however, the writing would still have been on the bathroom wall. Indeed, when St Augustine landed in Kent in 597 and began the process of converting the country to Christianity once and for all, his followers had no time for bathing. Theirs was an austere faith, which rejected all pleasures of the flesh, and the Romans had made no secret of the fact that pleasure was very much what bathing was about. The ethos of the thermae, notably at luxurious and fashionable bathing centres around the Empire such as Baden, Baden-Baden, Aix and Bath, ensured that, for Christians, every kind of bathing other than strictly religious ablutions was associated with iniquity – to the extent that a clean body represented an unclean mind.

As for the Anglo-Saxons, they appear to have rejected almost everything the Romans left behind. They did not even re-use the towns, let alone the baths. If they saw a hypocaust, they were probably baffled by it. The country villas lay in ruins, and the woods no longer resounded with cheery cries such as 'Quis meam strigilis utavit?'[1] or 'Ubi crepidae condemnatae meae sunt?'[2] Not surprisingly, the Anglo-Saxon standard of living remained far below that of the Romans. Even a royal palace, such as that of King Alfred at Cheddar in the ninth century, was lamentably short on creature comforts. Archaeologists believe that it may have had an outside loo, but it lacked the bathing facilities that would have been enjoyed by any middle-ranking Roman in his well-appointed villa over five centuries earlier. To be brutally frank, Alfred had no bath.

It is no exaggeration to say that for the best part of the Middle Ages bathing opportunities in England were extremely limited, arrangements positively medieval. The Vikings had brought very few civilized habits with them; the Normans – really just Christianized Vikings who had spent a few centuries in northern France limbering up for the conquest of England – were little better. They were certainly not in the business of making life agreeable for the vanquished Saxons. Even the Domesday Book, that extraordinary inventory of England's fixtures and fittings, fishponds and livestock etc, commissioned by William the Conqueror in 1085, has no chapter on baths.

Until about the twelfth century, ironically, such washing as did take place mostly did so, albeit in a strictly functional way, with no conceivable opportunity for enjoying it, in a religious setting. While the Church still frowned on public bathing, on the grounds that the public were sinful and that bathing clearly made them more so – something that was shortly to be confirmed in London – it was a different story, even in the darkest of ages, within the confines of the monastery. Here logic had clearly prevailed over the extremist teachings of St Paul, who held that bathing, marriage, sex – almost anything that you could think of – were sinful, but in the monasteries it had been recognized that the act of washing was in itself morally neutral. That being the case, a clean, refreshed body must be preferable to a tired, malodorous one, especially where large numbers of people were living at close quarters. As a result, not only did the monks wash their faces and hands daily, and their feet every Saturday, they would also have a bath – with soap – several times a year.

Now it was cleanliness that was being associated with godliness – even Popes agreed – and sophisticated systems of water supply, the first in England since Roman times, were introduced to promote it. By the twelfth century watercourses were being used to channel water from streams and springs up to three miles away. The water would then be conducted through lead pipes to the kitchen, bath-house and lavers – the stone troughs used for washing before and after meals – and beneath the latrines. Following the Black Death in 1348, from which a number of monasteries appeared to have been saved by their sanitary arrangements, the first attempts were made to improve London's sewage disposal system, which essentially consisted of the Fleet and Walbrook rivers.

These were good times to be a monk. If you were a Carthusian, indeed, you might well have had your own private water supply. There is evidence that the Charterhouse at Smithfield, in London, had gone to great lengths to provide such facilities by about 1435. The Carthusian way of life was less communal than that of other Orders. Instead of living in dormitories, the monks had their own individual cells, with a garden attached, and for the most part looked after themselves. A fifteenth-century document known as the 'Watercourse Parchment' shows that water was piped underground from springs on the slopes of Islington to a central conduit-house in the Great Cloister. From there pipes branched off to all sides of the cloister, supplying fresh water to the garden of each cell, and to the laundry, the kitchen and the brewhouse, and so on, as well as two local pubs. Almost exactly a century later, the Prior, John Houghton, and two other

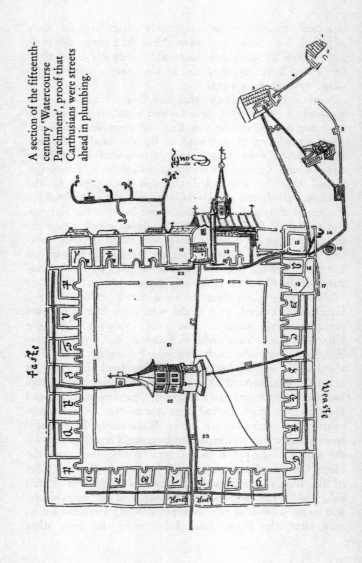

A section of the fifteenth-century 'Watercourse Parchment', proof that Carthusians were streets ahead in plumbing.

Carthusian Priors were the first to reject Henry VIII's Act of Supremacy and were barbarically executed. Who knows what further refinements in plumbing technology the Charterhouse might have developed had it not fallen victim to the Dissolution of the Monasteries which then followed?

For the record, after 70 years as a private residence in which it was turned into a sumptuous Elizabethan mansion, the former monastery became a charitable foundation with a double mission: as a Hospital, or home, for the well-connected but impoverished elderly, who were known as Brothers, and as a school for the children of people in similar straits. The Hospital remains; the school, having recaptured much of the spirit of its monastic past, before and after its move to Godalming in 1872, then achieved such footballing prowess, to add to its other distinctions, that in 1895 a team of Old Carthusians won the FA Cup. One wonders what the monk in his cell, silently washing his face in the laver filled from his garden tap, would have made of it all, had he been vouchsafed a glimpse of events to come.

Even better than having water on tap outside, some would say, is having a hot bath inside. That, in the last century or so before the Dissolution, is what many monks, such as Benedictines, had a right to expect. A cold bath might still be taken as a remedy for distracting thoughts, or as a penance, but hot water was now generally available – albeit probably not very often – for monks who trod the paths of righteousness. The bath itself would not have been a luxurious affair, simply a wooden tub, as the fixed, sunken bath was almost unheard of – though one was discovered in the courtyard of Kirkstall Abbey, in Yorkshire, with a stone for a plug – but no one was complaining about that. The drawback was that everyone used to share the same water, which would have been fine if you were one of the first, or at least could be some of the time. 'The first shall be last,' said Jesus, after all, 'and the last shall be first'

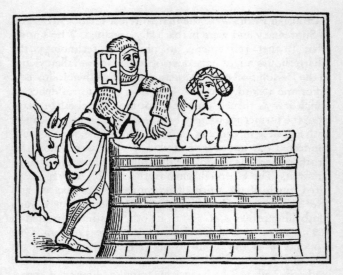

A thirteenth-century dalliance.

– but this never applied in the monastic bath-house. The prior or abbot used to be first in the tub, followed by the rest in descending order of seniority. What began as clean water must have have finished up as a cold and rather unpleasant *potage de moine* – bad luck on the unfortunate novice.

But at least they had baths. Others were not so lucky. As far as the poor were concerned, in England as in many other countries, there wasn't much chance of a bath, hot or cold, until the reforms of the mid-nineteenth century. Even for the rest, outside the monasteries, palaces and certain London establishments, a hot bath was a luxury in medieval England. For most, bathing consisted of sitting in a wooden tub of cold water, although enlarged or elongated versions existed here and there, enabling one to stretch out or entertain a friend. There are many charming medieval illustrations showing men and women bathing, singly or together, indoors or in the open air, with neither clothes nor embarrassment, and sometimes enjoying a meal or a drink as they do so. In one of them, from a thirteenth-century manuscript, a knight dabbles his fingers in the bath water of his mistress, who appears to be gossiping in the most natural way, or perhaps calling for refreshment. Baths must have been hard work, a deterrent unless you had plenty of domestic help. Piped water being a rarity, tubs would generally have had to be filled by hand – invariably in the case of hot water. It is hardly surprising, under the circumstances, that the bath did not enjoy cult status.

---

1. 'Who's been using my strigil?'
2. 'Where the devil are my slippers?'

5
Royal Pioneers

Although the bathing exploits of royalty have never borne much relation to the daily lives of their often grimy subjects, medieval England was blessed with several enterprising monarchs whose private contributions cannot be ignored. While nothing is known about the bathing habits of Richard the Lionheart, who may well have picked up some interesting ones from his Muslim opponents in the Holy Land, we do know something about his treacherous younger brother. King John, it is said, never let a month go by without taking a bath, and even if his was only a wooden one, that, as we have seen, was par for the course in thirteenth-century England.

John's son Henry, however, was an altogether more serious bather. This we can assume because there is an entry in the Westminster Chronicle for 1255 to the effect that he took delivery that year of a French-made bath, carved in stone in the shape of a peacock, 'covered all over with eyes like a real peacock, made of precious stones called pearls, gold, silver and saphires'. Presumably Henry either ordered this by messenger or had it sold to him by a representative armed with an illuminated catalogue or a golden tongue.

'And perhaps you would like to consider something for your mistress, Sire?'

'My mistress? Well, I don't know . . . Oh, you mean my wife – no, no indeed, she's perfectly happy with what she's got. Look, there she is outside. She's devoted to that tub. Unless you have any of those floating duck thingies?'

The year 1255 was a good one for imports, for it also saw the arrival in England of Eleanor of Castile, the young bride of the future Edward I. They had married the

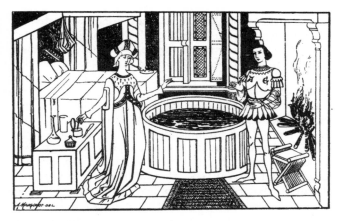

A royal bathing room.

previous year, when he was fourteen, she nine. Eleanor brought with her, if not a bath, then at least some sensible priorities, including a concern for a hygienic and comfortable lifestyle, possibly stemming from Moorish traditions. She is generally credited with popularizing the use in England not only of the bathtub but also of carpets. After a few years at Windsor she divided her time between various manors, including that of King's Langley. In 1278, by which time Edward was king and she had already borne nine children, she also took possession of Leeds Castle, in Kent. Edward now had a lot on his plate, including for the next five years the conquest of Wales (not a rewarding area as far as bathing amenities were concerned), and Eleanor got on with the job of turning King's Langley and Leeds into fit places in which to bring up a family. Several of her children had died in infancy, including the heir to the throne, and she did not want any repetition. At least one bath is known to have been installed at King's Langley, while at Leeds she went further. Records show that a consignment of 'one hundred Reigate stones' was delivered for the 'paving' of the 'King's bath'. This would be enough in itself to indicate that Edward managed to join Eleanor there from time to time – if we did not already know that between them in due course they contrived no fewer than sixteen children.

In fact the royal couple were devoted. The story goes that Eleanor once even saved Edward's life while they were in the Holy Land, presumably during the eighth Crusade of 1270. When he was stabbed with a poisoned dagger, she sucked the poison from his wound. After Eleanor died at Lincoln in 1290, aged 44, the grief-stricken Edward had 'Eleanor crosses' erected at stopping-places along the route by which her body was returned to London. The word 'charing' in Charing Cross, the most famous of these, stems from *chère reine*, meaning dear or beloved queen. After that he took it out on the Scots.

Eleanor's grandson Edward III was the next royal innovator in the bathroom. In addition to his substantial building projects at both Windsor Castle and the Palace of Westminster, where he completed St Stephen's Chapel and had a precursor of Big Ben mounted on a high tower facing the hall of Westminster, he did much to improve the living accommodation at the palace. In 1351, while the Hundred Years War was in its successful early phase, Edward installed England's first recorded baths with hot and cold piped water. His own bath, according to *King's Works*, had large bronze taps 'to bring hot and cold water in to the bath'. There is no evidence of any immediate trickle-down effect from this to improve the lives of his subjects, but in the area of public health Edward did, in the wake of the Black Death, take steps to improve the capital's abysmal sanitation system, which allowed most waste to run into the Fleet River. He gave orders for the river to be cleared, for no more privies to be built over it, and for cesspits to be used instead. In the long run this action was probably more valuable to his country than all the victories then being won in France. (His son, who was responsible for many of them, was also called Edward, but not many people know this, because this fiery character regarded bathing as something for lily-livered civilians and went down in history as the Black Prince.)

At the end of the fourteenth century there were even baths at the Tower of London. It was there, on the eve of the coronation of Henry IV in 1399, that the bathtub suddenly shot to fame by taking on a unique and unexpected ceremonial role. It appears that about 50 followers of the Duke of Lancaster, as he then was, were induced to undergo purifying baths in the White Tower, and that Henry conferred on them an entirely new order of knighthood which inevitably became known as the Order of the Bath. Then, after a night of vigil in St John's Chapel, these new Knights of the Bath accompanied him to Westminster for the coronation. The oddest thing about the episode is that the candidates actually received their accolade in the bath. No one knows why.

Thereafter the ceremony took place whenever a king was to be crowned, and became highly formalized. Under the direction of two 'esquires of honour grave', the prospective knight would be shaved, undressed and placed in a bath 'hung within and without with linen and rich cloths'. Seated in the bath, he would receive instruction from two venerable knights about the Order and other matters chivalric, and have water poured over him. After being put in a bed to dry, he would be dressed in a robe with a hood and led to the chapel. There, with his sword and shield placed in front of him, and the two esquires and the priest in attendance, he would spend the night in contemplation and prayer. In the morning, all sin having been removed from his soul, he was ready to be elevated to the knighthood.

The Order of the Bath was discontinued after the coronation of Charles II, but reinstated in 1725 by George I.

Since 1847 it has included civilians and, since 1970, even women. The Order now has three grades: Knights Companions (CB), Knights Commanders (KCB) and Knights of the Grand Cross (GCB). Their relative costs are a closely guarded secret.

More significantly, the knighthood is now conferred without recourse to the Tower of London *or even to a bath*. It is too soon to say whether the quality and performance of today's knights have been impaired as a result, but one cannot help fearing for the future. Nor can one help regretting the passing of such a colourful piece of ceremonial, especially one whose symbolism speaks to us so much more clearly than other absurd rituals which have mysteriously survived. Its loss is all the sadder in view of its excellent televisual possibilities:

'Welcome back, and we're going straight over to the White Tower, where earlier this evening we saw Jeffrey Archer, soon to be Sir Jeffrey, coming through the purifying bath with flying colours. Now I'm hearing that he's run into a spot of bother. Let's find out how he's getting on with that tricky silent vigil . . .'

6
Steamy Stuff

While the knight dallied at his lady's tub and the abbot turned his mind to plumbing, something risqué was going on in London. As in cities all over Europe, the general public were starting to enjoy an age of steam.

The steam or vapour bath goes right back into the mists of time. It probably existed long before anyone thought of running a liquid one. It appears that some kind of basic vapour bath was used in Asia in prehistoric times and gradually made its way westwards to Syria, Greece, Russia and Finland. We know little about its early forms, however, because prehistoric periods are notoriously ill-documented. One assumes that it consisted of nothing more complicated than chucking a bit of water onto hot stones in an enclosed space such as a hut. That, in fact, is roughly how the Russian vapour bath remained until the twentieth century.

Elsewhere it developed along independent lines. The Syrians built purely hot-air bath-houses, while the Greeks put the emphasis jointly on cold-water baths and gymnastic and intellectual exercise. They thought heat was for wimps, but later saw the error of their ways, as did the Romans. When the Roman Empire encompassed Syria, the conquerors' version of bathing largely eclipsed the local one, and smaller versions of their multi-roomed thermae were built. When the Roman influence waned, however, Syrian bath-house design evolved again, with less emphasis on the cold and tepid rooms, and more on the warm and hot ones.

It was this composite of the Syrian and Roman bath-house that was in place when Islam expanded into the area in the seventh century AD. The Muslims could see a useful purpose in the thermae, but not for gymnastics or debates.

They were not going to be swimming either, so the pool could go, along with the palestra and the library. They preserved the arrangement of cool, warm and hot rooms, but the laconicum, which previously provided dry heat, now became a steam room, and instead of exercising, bathers were pummelled and massaged. The biggest difference was that there was no more bathing in water. It was better, according to Islamic belief, to sweat one's impurities away than to soak in them. Meanwhile the mood of the building was also transformed. Whereas the thermae had high vaulted roofs, with enormous windows letting in plenty of light, the *hammam*, as the Islamic bath-house was called, had lower roofs in the form of cupolas. The atmosphere inside became dark, restful and religious.

In cities all across the Islamic world, from the Middle East to North Africa and Spain, the hammam provided a form of relaxation compatible with the Islamic faith and became the chief meeting-place for ordinary Muslims of both sexes – though not together. It was to travel all over Europe in the Middle Ages, and in the eighteenth and nineteenth centuries would enjoy brief vogues in the West as the Turkish bath, before itself having to give way, even in the Middle East, to the ubiquitous Western bathtub.

Various forms of vapour bath also existed independently in other parts of the world. In Mexico, for example, long before the Europeans came, a sweating bath was used to treat fevers, rheumatism and poisonous bites. The bather would be enclosed in a kind of sunken oven, into which steam would be forced by pouring water onto stones made red hot by a stove right next to the oven. Enveloped in steam, the bather would apply healing herbs to the parts affected. North American Indian tribes are known to have contrived a vapour bath inside a lodge or wigwam. Here the bather would sit suspended in a basket contraption containing herbs; red-hot stones, heated in a furnace outside, would be brought in and placed beneath it and

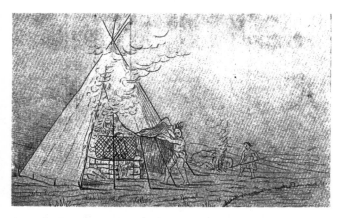

An early American vapour bath.

splashed with water to produce steam. This would often be followed by a plunge into a cold river or lake, or, as in Russia, a roll in the snow. The Russians also favoured beating each other with twigs – and still do.

It is said that in ancient times even the Scots and Irish discovered how reviving steam could be. The Ancient Britons apparently never did. Confronted with the hot springs of Bath, they could think of no use for them. Even when the Romans helpfully gave a 400-year demonstration it just didn't seem to stick, and after they had left, the springs reverted to marshland for approximately seven centuries.

It was not until the twelfth century that the vapour bath was seen again in England, and then it was imported from abroad. It was brought back either by travellers returning from the East or, as is generally supposed, by Crusaders returning from Palestine. Typically, having gone there for something completely different, they came back saying, 'Look at these wonderful carpets – they are for walking on.

They'll help to keep your feet warm in winter. Yes, and there's another thing we have to try. The heathens have got these amazing rooms which they fill with vapour, all you need is a bucket of water and a few stones which you heat on the fire, and you get all hot and steamy and sweat like mad and afterwards you feel great – oh and it makes you clean too.' At this point the wife probably said, 'I don't like the sound of that, but I'll take a dozen carpets.'

In fact vapour baths quickly became extremely popular, with men and women, at a time when no other form of bathing was. In London in particular they caught on in a big way, and the hammam or *bagnio* – from the Italian – became the latest social centre. Unfortunately there seems to be something about massage and saunas, because it was not long before the exquisite Islamic custom began to be used by Londoners as an excuse for debauchery. Hammam, bagnio, hothouse, stew – it had many names but one particular function which, despite all the steam, was crystal clear: it was a brothel. Having been God-fearing and dirty, medieval Cockneys became debauched and clean. From the churches came a muttering which quickly grew louder – loudest of all from St Paul's, no doubt – and the message was: 'I told you so.'

Henry II tried legislation to curb these dens of vice, but such was their popularity that they survived nearly another 400 years. During the reign of Richard II there were eighteen of them in Southwark alone. Something more drastic needed to be done. Eventually it was.

7
Renaissance of Hot Water

The steam-bath vogue was a pan-European phenomenon which gave a boost to bathing in general. What people enjoyed and wanted, particularly in cold northern climates, was heat, and the fifteenth century saw an unprecedented rise in the number of bathing establishments offering hot-water baths as well as steam rooms. They were sociable places, where those who could afford it went not just to wash, but to relax, talk and enjoy themselves in a deliciously warm environment.

The most famous bathing centre in Renaissance Europe was Baden, near Zurich in Switzerland, whose hot springs had been greatly prized by the Romans. The fashionable Italian writer Poggio Bracciolini visited Baden in 1414 and could hardly believe his eyes:

The baths are altogether 30 in number. Of these, two only are public baths, which are exposed to view on every side, and are frequented by the lower orders of people, of all ages, and of each sex. Here the males and females, entertaining no hostile dispositions towards each other, are separated only by a simple railing. It is a droll sight to see decrepit old women and blooming maidens stepping into the water, and exposing their charms to the profane eyes of the men ... The baths belonging to the private houses are very neat. They too are common to males and females, who are separated by a partition. In this partition, however, there are low windows, through which they can see and converse with, and touch each other, and also drink together; all which circumstances are common occurrences ... As the ladies go in and out of the water, they expose to view a considerable portion of their persons; yet there are no door-keepers, or even doors, nor do they entertain the least idea of anything approaching to indelicacy.

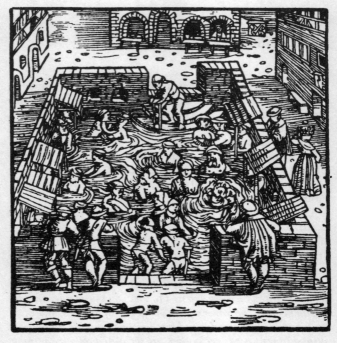

Taking to the water at the medicinal bathing resort of Plombière-les-Bains, in the Vosges.

Many of the baths have a common passage for the two sexes, which circumstance very frequently occasions very curious encounters. The men wear only a pair of drawers. The women are clad in linen vests, which are however slashed in the sides, so that they neither cover the neck, the breast, nor the arms of the wearer . . . As I only bathed twice a day, I spent my leisure time in witnessing this curious spectacle, visiting the other baths, and causing the girls to scramble for money and nosegays; for there was no opportunity for reading or studying.

We don't know what Poggio came to Baden to study, but the above extracts from his long and detailed description of the baths suggest that he had found a subject close to his heart.

The Church, as ever, frowned on such goings-on, and on public baths in general. Famous centres such as Baden and Bath – which, as we shall see, was also in full swing once again – were able to resist religious opposition. Others survived by enforcing just enough discipline; the key to acceptability lay in strict segregation of the sexes. In Germany, where steam baths were especially popular, discipline was predictably good. The bathers in Nuremberg observed in 1496–7 by Dürer, for example, seem to be well under control, though with the media present they may have been told to be on their best behaviour. Some bathing places managed to prohibit the clergy from entering – a novel way of reducing the number of complaints. (There may even be a lesson here for the 1990s. Expressions of outrage over the content of television programmes would surely decline if those encumbered with a moral sense were unable to obtain a TV licence.)

The less orderly establishments, chiefly the urban steam baths, or stews, where prostitutes plied their trade, came in for increasingly fierce denunciations. Eventually the moral majority carried the day, the authorities agreeing that these stews were no better than cess-pits, and several monarchs felt obliged to step in. The first casualties were the Moorish baths in Granada. The Moors were not even behaving badly – they were just Moorish – but King Alfonso decided that the best way to teach them a lesson for persisting in being heathen was to close their baths. Such was the strength of feeling of this master psychologist that even private baths were forbidden them. Those must have been difficult times for the committed Moorish bather. In France in 1538, François I went one better by having the stews of Paris demolished. In England at about the same

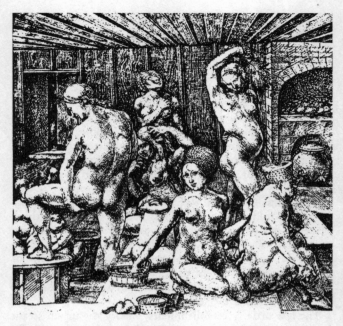

The Women's Bath, by Albrecht Dürer. Nuremberg, 1496.

time, Henry VIII, not content with dissolving the monasteries, issued such strict regulations that the stews were effectively banned. All that remained were highly respectable bath-houses – dull but correct, as befitted the reign of such a stickler for form.

This is precisely the kind of action which helped give Henry his possibly rather unjustified reputation as a petulant, bullying king, a bad husband and very probably a non-bather to boot. (Curiously, he is nevertheless one of the most popular figures among English monarchs.) Now in any case this verdict is sure to be revised, at least as regards the last charge, for in April 1996 the British

Museum made a startling announcement. It concerned a collection of tiles which had been recovered during the excavation of the site of the Palace of Whitehall in 1939, and which the museum had now had time to evaluate. They were, said an excited curator, almost certainly the remains of a sumptuous, state-of-the-art Turkish bath dating from Henry's reign. It was safe to say that the king had had what amounted to a fitted bathroom, containing a large sunken stone bath and a twelve-foot-high wood-fired stove of classical design, decorated with tiles bearing heraldic symbols and continental-style grotesques – 'very much the latest thing in interior decoration'. Of course there is no way of knowing whether Henry actually used the bathroom or had it chiefly for show. It could be that he had heard reports of something similar belonging to his French pen-pal François I, with whom he had a cordial if somewhat competitive relationship, and simply wanted to upstage him. We will never know, but in view of the bad press that Henry has had over the years, one is inclined to give him the benefit of the doubt.

Be that as it may, having declared himself supreme head of the Church, dissected alive a number of leading churchmen and thus cocked an almighty snook at the Pope, poor Henry would still have been distraught if he could have seen the pontiff's bathroom. The cylindrical Castel St Angelo in Rome, originally built as the tomb of the Emperor Hadrian but later converted into a fortress, does not have the air of a luxurious papal dwelling; in fact it looks more like a medieval bathtub. Within, however, Pope Clement VII had apartments containing possibly the most ornate bathroom ever built. Frescoes covered the walls, which in the old Roman style contained hot-air flues to make his *stufetta* (literally, 'little stew') something like a caldarium, if not a laconicum. The bath itself was made of marble, and hot and cold water were available therein at the touch of the papal toes. Saints Paul and Francis would have had a fit.

They would have been more concerned, however, had reports reached them of the orgiastic bathing activities at the Vatican. Something of the tenor of the age can be gauged from the notorious graffito found there – albeit long since erased, its authenticity in any case angrily rejected by Vatican historians – of which a rough translation is given below.

'A voluptuous monk from Milan
Came to Rome with a perilous plan:
"It's a risk to take,
But I try to make
A cardinal sin – if I can."'

Apart from Henry VIII, the Tudors seem to have made little contribution to the progress of the bath. Edward VI never really had a chance, being cut off in his prime, and his half-sister Mary was too busy burning Protestant bishops to give it much thought. It is therefore a relief to be able to report that Queen Elizabeth at least had a bath. It was called Queen Elizabeth's Bath and was a fine, square, stone-built affair with stepped sides, under a vaulted brick roof. It was situated at Charing Cross, which cannot have been all that convenient since the Queen's main residences were the palaces of Richmond, Greenwich and Havering, in Essex. One wonders whether she used it very often. Apart from anything else, it was a public bath, and while Bess was renowned for having the common touch, even she must have drawn the line somewhere.

Much of the Queen's time in any case was spent on the road, on her famous 'progresses' around the country, inspecting some of the great houses that her courtiers were so keen on building. A visit from Elizabeth and her retinue placed a severe strain on her host's finances – and on his drains. However, she was normally considerate, or squeamish, enough to move on after a couple of days, before the smell became intolerable.

One aristocrat who dreaded her visit was Sir John

Thynne, whose descendants would be Marquesses of Bath, and whose grandiose building project at Longleat in Wiltshire was arousing everyone's curiosity. For a while he managed to put her off with excuses – being able to say that his house had burnt down must have seemed like a godsend – but eventually even he had to give way. The visit presumably went well, because Sir John got the royal thumbs-up in a note from the court: 'Thanks be to God, Her Majesty is well returned with good health and great liking her entertainment in ye West parts, and namely [especially], at your house, which twice sithence to myself, and the last Sonday to my Lady's grace, she greatly commended.'

If the Elizabethan age was not a golden one for the bath, it was a close thing for the loo. Another royal thank-you letter which one wishes had survived is the one she may or may not have sent – perhaps even written herself, as the matter was delicate – to another Sir John, her godson Sir John Harington. This was a man of vision who, not content with designing the first ever flushing water closet and describing its workings in a witty and scandalously satirical book about sewage disposal, actually presented one of the prototypes to Her Majesty for use at the Palace of Richmond. (Very likely she used to tell him when he was a child that the nicest possible present would be 'something you've made yourself' – if so, this time he had really excelled himself.) The upshot, however, is a mystery, for nothing seems to have come of this apparent breakthrough. All we know is that it was almost two hundred years before the next flushing loo came along. So what happened? It may simply be, as historians have assumed, that the Queen looked into Sir John's device and could see nothing in it, but one cannot help feeling that something must have gone horribly wrong. Probably she either failed to assemble the contraption correctly or didn't feel that it was worth having Richmond Palace plumbed for so small a thing . . . Or perhaps she just couldn't be bothered to read the small print. In which case she may have treated the water closet like her much-loved close stool (a glorified chamber pot which was basically just a padded bucket) – and been disappointed with the outcome.

'Deare John,' she would perhaps have written (making this the original 'Dear John' letter), 'Wee are pursuaded thatte thye late gift of the streaming Place of Easement was intended loyally; howsomever it hath notte pleased usse, for it hath splashed our hinder partes and mired our carpette. The inventor of this foule Contraptioun should therefore goe back toe his draughtsman's boarde or better still get himselfe toe another Countrie . . .' We do know that Sir John Harington was indeed banished from court at about that time, and while all this is speculation, it may well explain everything. Whatever the truth of the matter, one feels that in one way or another Elizabeth let the side down badly, depriving her country of a potential jewel, if not in its crown, then under its bottom.

After that detour, or P-trap as we say in plumbing circles, we return refreshed to the bath. The truth about Queen Elizabeth's bathing habits is that we don't know anything about them, beyond the fact that she was reported by an admiring contemporary to be in the habit of taking a bath every month, 'whether she needed it or no'. This double-edged testimonial probably tells us rather more about the tenor of the age than does the bare fact that there were 'bathing-rooms' at Windsor Castle in her time, one of which was 'wainscotted with looking-glass'. Another clue is that there are scarcely any references to bathing in the works of Shakespeare, which contain almost everything else. What few there are mostly refer to hands being bathed in blood, which is beyond our remit.

In some respects, it seems, the reign of Queen Elizabeth I was a disappointment. To be sure, there was much technological progress, notably in the field of architecture. Fine new mansions were going up all over the country, often to designs by Italian architects and with state-of-the-art furnishings and decor in wood and plaster by Italian craftsmen. However, there is little evidence of bathrooms, Italianate or otherwise, featuring in their plans, and the blossoming science of hydraulics was mainly being used to pump water into fountains, cascades and joke statues and ornaments which sprayed the unwary passer-by, rather than to where it was really needed. The bathroom, where it existed at all, tended to be an alcove with a bathtub concealed behind a curtain. Otherwise you just dragged your tub over to the fire on which you laboriously heated the water. The only concessions to hedonism were the sprinkling of fragrant herbs on the water and the use of scented soaps.

A few hopeful signs can be seen, however, in the area of public health. For one thing, some of Elizabeth's subjects were at last cleaning their teeth, using the new tooth powder which had just arrived – but it can't have been easy, because the toothbrush hadn't. Tooth cleaning, fortunately, did not require large quantities of water, which for many people were still not available. Here and there, however, progress was even being made in the provision of clean water. In Devon, a highly successful project was conceived and carried out by none other than Sir Francis Drake. Taking time off from exploring, buccaneering and tormenting the Spaniards, he constructed a winding channel, eighteen miles long, to carry water down a gentle incline from Dartmoor to Plymouth. (Had he chosen a more direct route, it would have come with too much of a rush.) Sir Francis had his private motives, to do with the servicing of his fleet, but it was a notable public improvement. One hopes that the people of Plymouth, who already doubtless thanked the Lord for the food they were about to receive, thereafter uttered a word or two of gratitude to Sir Francis for the bath . . .

In London, too, new conduits were built to bring water in from the countryside. The need had been recognized at last. Indeed, as early as 1539, following devastating outbreaks of the plague, Sir Thomas Elyot had published his *Castel of Helth*, in which he blamed the rapid spread of the disease on poor living conditions, especially on 'much people in small room living uncleanly and slutishly'. At least the connection was now being made, even if it would be a long time before anything substantial was done about it. In fact, the city's sanitary conditions would get much worse before they got better, and the shortage of clean water would remain a major cause of Britain's poor standards of public hygiene and her relative failure as a bathing nation. From this point of view the Renaissance, in Britain, was a bit of a flash in the pan.

8
Little Dark Age

English attitudes to personal hygiene in the seventeenth century are best summed up by a remark made by Lady Mary Wortley Montague when a French visitor commented on the filthy state of her hands. 'Madame,' Lady Mary replied, 'if you think these are dirty, you should see my feet!' Although her one-liner sounds rather modern – history does not relate whether she went in for body-piercing or recreational drug-taking, but one wouldn't be at all surprised – she was very much a child of her time. Her contemporaries were positively proud to be dirty. There was no need to be clean, they seem to have decided, when they had such fine clothes and fragrant perfumes. Besides, they were now the proud users of underwear and even nightwear, and all these could be changed if necessary, which seemed to obviate the necessity to go through the rigmarole of washing the body.

Technology, perversely, provided another excuse for washing even less than before. The fork was now in fairly general use (the table fork, that is – farmers and gardeners had been forking for years), and now that people were no longer putting their fingers into the same bowl, as well as into their mouths, they obviously felt no need to wash their hands before and after meals. Thus the laver was redundant and in the dining-room there was a failure even to maintain medieval standards of hygiene.

Remarkably, one of the worst culprits in hygienic matters seems to have been that carefree monarch Charles II. He and his courtiers did not care where they relieved themselves, and felt free to use any convenient corner or the privacy of a curtain. The diarist Anthony à Wood was unamused by the aftermath of a visit to Oxford by Charles and his gang in 1665: 'Though they were neat and gay in their apparell, yet they were very nasty and beastly, leaving at their departure their excrements in every corner, in chimneys, studies, colehouses, cellers. Rude, rough, whoremongers; vaine, empty, careless.' In Charles's defence it should be noted that there is documentary evidence of work being done on a bathing room in Whitehall Palace in about 1670. It is not clear whether he was installing a new one or altering an existing one, but the possibility exists, in the latter case, that he was making improvements to the Turkish bath of Henry VIII.

Amid all these sins of omission and commission it is pleasant to be able to acclaim at least one genuine hero of this benighted age. John Aubrey relates that early in the century the philosopher and one-time Lord Chancellor Francis Bacon lived so nobly at Gorhambury, St Albans, that 'his Watermen were more imployed by Gentlemen than any other, even the King's'. Furthermore, when Bacon built Verulam House nearby, he incorporated 'two Bathing-roomes or Stuffes, whither his Lordship retired afternoons as he saw cause'. Perhaps he was influenced by the area's Roman past, for these sound very much like hothouses. In his posthumous *Historie of Life and Death*, Bacon wrote at length about the virtues of bathing (for which he had plenty of time following his banishment from Parliament for bribery), and recommended the following procedure:

Common mollifying, softening Baths doe rather draw than soften, and loosen rather than harden the Body . . . First, before bathing, rub and anoint the Body with Oyle, and Salves, that the Baths moistening heate and virtue may penetrate into the body, and not the liquors watery part: then sit two houres in the Bath; after Bathing wrap the Body in a seare-cloth made of Masticke, Myrrh, Pomander, and Saffron, for staying the perspiration or breathing of the pores, untill the softening of the body, having layne thus in

seare-cloth 24 hours, bee growne solid and hard. Lastly,
with an oyntment of Oyle, Salt, and Saffron, the seare-cloth
being taken off, anoint the body.

Interestingly, soap is not included in the operation,
which, it has been pointed out, would have taken, allowing
time for undressing and dressing, rubbing and anointing,
about 27 hours. Disappointingly, an ungrateful nation
seems to have spurned this sound advice.

The diary of Samuel Pepys, generally the most reliable
barometer for the Restoration climate, contains a couple of
revealing references to bathing. Pepys, who seems to have
enjoyed the use of a close stool but not that of a bathroom,
refers in somewhat ambiguous terms to his wife having on
one occasion taken a bath: 'My wife busy in going with her
woman to the hot house to bathe herself, after her long
being within doors in the dirt, so that she now pretends to a
resolution of being hereafter very clean. How long it will
hold I can guess.' The tone is clearly sceptical, but the
implication could be either that he was himself a committed
bather, or that he doubted whether bathing was ever likely
to catch on. One leans towards the latter when one reads his
glowing account of a visit to the house of a Mr Thomas
Povey in 1664: '. . . his room floored above with woods of
several colours . . . his grotto and vault, with his bottles of
wine, and a well therein to keep them cool; his furniture of
all sorts; his bath at the top of the house, good pictures,
and his manner of eating and drinking; do surpass all that
ever I did see of one man in all my life.' The bath is the
most surprising item for the period and is probably what
most tickled his fancy in this state-of-the-art household. It
would not, incidentally, have been plumbed in, except perhaps to a tank in the roof, as water was not pumped to
upper floors for at least another century. Mr Povey's water
would have had to be carried upstairs, either by watermen
or his own servants. This is one reason why private baths
in Restoration England were so few and far between.

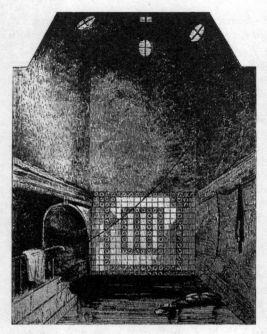

Queen Anne's Bath.

Towards the end of the seventeenth century London had a number of public baths, of which the most famous was in Endell Street, St Giles's, near the junction with Long Acre. Later reputed to be a favourite resort of Queen Anne, it became known as Queen Anne's Bath, but was constructed well before her time. It was a little plunge bath, supplied by a powerful spring with cold water which was supposed to bring relief from rheumatic complaints.

The earth was dug out round the spring, and over it was built a lofty domed apartment, about 12 feet by 10 feet in area, and about 24 feet in height from the floor to the crown of the roof. The floor of the bath was paved with squares of marble, alternately black and white, and the sides were covered with Dutch tiles, some white, and some with blue-and-white designs upon them. To secure the bath from leakage more effectually, sheets of copper were inserted under the flooring and wall-tiles.

There was a dressing-room near at hand, from whence was a descent of several steps to the bath. Light was admitted to this room by narrow skylights, and to the bath by means of a narrow window in the crown of the roof, and four small circular windows around it. Upon one side of the bath there was a platform from which bathers could plunge into the water . . .

Just nearby in Long Acre life was considerably hotter – at the Duke's Bagnio. Towards the end of the century, following experiments in Constantinople by intrepid travellers, the much-maligned 'stew', now known either as a 'bagnio' or a 'hummum' (from the Turkish *hammam*), made a spectacular reappearance in London as an exotic imported luxury. The most fashionable were the Royal Bagnio, opened in 1679, and the Duke's Bagnio, which was described by Samuel Haworth as

a stately oval edifice, with a cupola roof, in which are round glasses to let in light. The cupola is supported by eight columns, between which and the sides is a sumptuous walk, arched over with brick. The bagnio is paved with marble, and has a marble table; the sides are covered with white gully-tiles, and within the wall are ten seats, such as are in the baths at Bath. There are also fourteen niches in the walls, in which are placed so many fonts or basins, with cocks over them of hot or cold water . . . Adjoining to the bagnio, there are four little round rooms, about eight feet over, which are made for degrees of heat, some being hotter, others colder, as persons can best bear and are pleased to use. These rooms are also covered with cupolas, and their walls with gully-tiles.

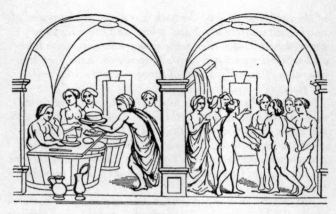

An all-girls room in a seventeenth-century bagnio.

After an hour or more of sweating, the bather would then be taken in hand by a 'rubber', who pulled and stretched the joints, provided a thorough wash, and then, in a cooler room, 'rubs his body all over with a hair-chamelot glove, which gently scratcheth the skin, and is exceedingly pleasant to the senses. After he hath continued this pleasant sort of friction for some time, more or less, as the person desires it, he fetcheth a basin of perfumed lather, with which he washes the body all over.'

Far from being the licenced brothels of old, the new bagnios were luxurious establishments, which claimed to have a curative function and which were the height of fashion for a short time – until they were perceived to spread more diseases than they cured, often of the venereal kind, and to have descended into . . . unlicenced brothels. With disapproval coming from both religious and medical quarters, their days were numbered. For a short time, however, the combination of bath-house and whorehouse was hugely successful. In commercial terms the connection was too good not to be made. Whereas a pillar of the community might have baulked at announcing that he was 'just popping down to the brothel', it was quite a lot easier to sigh that it had been a long day and he was going over to freshen up. Once the cats were out of the bagnio, the desire for freshening up among Londoners was generally less urgent.

The bagnio had yet another lease of life in the late eighteenth century – with similar results. The description of the bagnio experience provided by Casanova, who visited London in about 1765, is a model of succinctness: 'I also visited the bagnios, where a rich man can sup, bathe and sleep with a fashionable courtesan, of which species there are many in London. It makes a magnificent debauch and only costs six guineas.' As the great lover would have said, had he been French, '*Plus ça change . . .*'

It is difficult to know why, bagnios apart (and Bath apart – to which we shall come), the seventeenth century was quite such a wasted one. Some have put it down to the Reformation and, in particular, the Puritan idea of the body being unworthy of consideration, the naked body horribly sinful. It became such an obsession, they claim, that everything connected with the body needed to be swept under the carpet. This may be going a bit far – though we have seen that some Stuarts were not averse to using the curtains – and one is reluctant to blame everything on religion, whether established or non-conformist. It may be that the abhorrence for what was natural was itself just a natural phenomenon, like the change in the world's climate which led to the period between the fifteenth and eighteenth centuries being known as the Little Ice Age. Perhaps this dismal spell in bathing history should just be written off as a Little Dark Age.

9
The Glory that was Bath

The one place in England where bathing was regularly practised was Bath itself. For the hot spring revered by the Romans had been rediscovered in medieval times, and as early as the thirteenth century Bath was once again a place of pilgrimage for those suffering from rheumatism and many other complaints, including, it must be said, boredom. Bath shines like a beacon through almost the whole of English bathing history, but almost independently of it, as a glorious exception, for people came to bathe at Bath who bathed nowhere else. Until the eighteenth century, when bathing became more or less incidental to the city's other attractions, the motive for coming was purely medicinal.

The Tudor travel writer John Leland visited Bath in the 1540s, and his *Itinerary* contains a detailed description of the bathing arrangements, of whose flavour these extracts provide an interesting, if not altogether mouth-watering sample:

There are two springs of hot water in the WSW part of the town. The larger of them is called the Cross Bath, because it has a cross erected in the centre of it. This bath is much frequented by people suffering from diseases such as leprosy, pox, skin complaints, and severe pain. It is pleasantly warm, and there are eleven or twelve stone arches along the sides where people may shelter from the rain. This bath has alleviated many skin conditions and pains. Two hundred feet away there is another bath, called the Hot Bath, because when people first encounter it they think that it will scald them, but once their bodies have become acclimatized to it, it is more bearable and agreeable. It covers a smaller area than the Cross Bath, and has only seven arches along the wall . . .

The King's Bath is very fine and large. It stands almost in the centre of the town, and at the west end of the cathedral church. The bath and its precinct are surrounded by a high stone wall. Around the edge of the bath itself is a low wall, into which is built an arcade of thirty-two niches, in which men and women can stand privately. It is to this bath that the gentry resort . . .

The water in the baths is the colour of deep blue seawater, and it churns continually like a boiling pot, giving off a somewhat unpleasant and sulphurous odour . . . In all three baths it is plainly visible how the water bubbles up from the springs.

The amenities may have been somewhat primitive in Tudor times, but better things were at hand. The catalyst for the resurgence of this Roman oasis as a fashionable bathing resort was a visit by, of all people, a Stuart. James I's wife, Anne of Denmark, came to Bath in 1616 and she had such an unpleasant experience that for a moment the whole future of Bath can be said to have hung in the balance. She was happily bathing in the King's Bath when, according to Richard Warner's *History of Bath* (1801), 'there arose from the bottom of the cistern, just by the side of her Majesty, a flame of fire, like a candle, which had no sooner ascended to the top of the water than it spread itself upon the surface into a large circle of light, and then became extinct.' The Queen, not unreasonably taking the view that she had come to be gently simmered, not flambéed, was greatly put out – and got out – and all the Queen's doctors and all the Queen's friends couldn't get Anne to go back in again. Eventually, however, she was game for more and tried a different bath, a newly built one which had no hot spring of its own and therefore no such tricks to play. This was a complete success and was known thereafter as the Queen's Bath.

Suddenly, Bath was where everyone wanted to be seen, ill or not, and such was the enthusiasm for bathing that things seem to have got a bit out of hand. The architect John Wood, to whom Bath owes many of its finest buildings, was later to write: 'The Baths were like so many Bear Gardens, and Modesty was entirely shut out of them; People of both Sexes bathing by Day and Night naked; and Dogs, cats, and even human creatures were hurl'd over the rails into the water, while People were bathing in it.'

Here at last was something a Roman could relate to – but you can't please everyone. Modesty is a dull girl, who never has been much fun in the bath, but she should not have been shut out. That's obvious. All she wanted was something a bit more salubrious. In the event, it wasn't long before she had the baths all to herself.

Charles II was not deterred by Bath's reputation and turned up in 1663 with his court and his wife, Catherine of Braganza. The object was to find a cure for her sterility, and huge crowds cheered them on their way to the baths. The royal couple took to the waters with high hopes – but it was not to be. As a later Bath historian, R.A.L. Smith, neatly put it, 'the main purpose of their visit was not realized. Catherine could find no cure and her husband's paternal instincts found expression elsewhere'. A few years later Queen Mary, the wife of James II, came to Bath with similar intent, and on this occasion by contrast the experience was a complete success – the 'fecundating springs' bringing her barrenness to a happy end. Whether or not the experience of either Queen had much to do with the waters is a moot point. Either way, Bath never looked back.

By the turn of the century, even the tone had improved, for it is clear from her own account that no animals were thrown when, for example, the distinguished traveller and diarist Celia Fiennes tried the baths in 1695. Here she is in the Cross Bath:

When you would walk about the bath I use to have a woman guide or two to Lead me for the water is so strong it

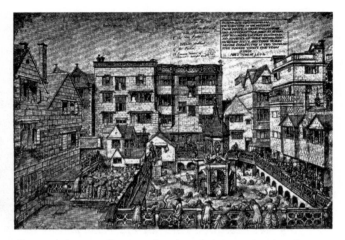

Thomas Johnson's drawing of Bath in the 1670s, showing the King's Bath on the right, the Queen's Bath on the left.

will quickly tumble you down, and then you have two of the men guides goes at a distance about the bath to Cleare the way. At the sides of the Arches are rings that you may hold by and so walke a little way, but the springs bubbles up so fast and so strong and are so hot up against the bottoms of ones feete, Especially in that they Call the Kitching in the bath, which is a great Cross with seates in the middle and many hot springs riseth there. The Kings bath is very large, as large as the rest put together, in it is the hot pumpe that persons are pumpt at for lameness or on their heads for palsyes . . . The Ladyes goes into the bath with Garments made of a fine yellow canvas, which is stiff and made large with great sleeves like a parsons gown; the water fills it up so that its borne off that your shape is not seen, it does not cling close as other linning, which Lookes sadly in the poorer sort that go in their own linning. The Gentlemen have drawers and wastcoates of the same sort of canvas, this is the best linning, for the bath water will Change any other yellow. When you go out of the bath you go within a doore that leads to Steps which you ascend by degrees that are in the water, then the doore is shut which shuts down into the water a good way, so you are in a private place where you still ascend severall more steps and let your Canvass drop of by degrees into the water, which your women guides take off, and the meane tyme your maides flings a garment of flannell made like a Nightgown with great sleeves over your head, and the guides take the taile and so pulls it on you Just as you rise the steps, and your other garment drops off so you are wrapped up in the flannell and your nightgown on the top, and your slippers and so you are set in Chaire which is brought into the roome which are called slips, and there are Chimney's in them, you may have fires. These are in severall parts of the sides of the bath for the Conveniency of persons going in and out of the bath decently . . .

They seem to have had everything covered, so it was clearly safe for Modesty to go back in the water, albeit without her maid, Syntax, who would follow on later.

Queen Anne visited Bath in 1702 – also the year in which Beau Nash first arrived – and in the decades which followed the city changed out of all recognition. As Master of Ceremonies, Nash not only laid on first-class balls and other entertainments but drew up and enforced such strict rules of etiquette that people of fashion, including royalty, knew that they could safely patronize the baths, the concert hall and the Pump Room without any risk of exposure to impropriety – let alone furry missiles.

Although the baths were still the city's chief *raison d'être* at the start of the eighteenth century, they were not to be for very much longer. As early as the 1720s Daniel Defoe was noting, in his *Tour Through the Whole Island of Great Britain*: 'The bathing is more a sport and diversion than a physical prescription for health.' He also observed:

'. . . there are many more come to drink the waters, than to bathe in them; nor are the cures they perform this way, less valuable than the outward application; especially in colics, ill digestion, and scorbutic distempers.' Increasingly bathing was taking its place as just one of Bath's attractions and was described by Oliver Goldsmith as 'no unpleasing method of passing away an hour or so'. This would take place between six and nine o'clock in the morning, after which came the serious business of the day:

The amusement of bathing is immediately succeeded by a general assembly of people at the pump-room; some for pleasure, and some to drink the hot waters. Three glasses at three different times is the usual portion for every drinker; and the intervals between every glass are enlivened by the harmony of a small band of music, as well as by the conversation of the gay, the witty, or the forward. From the pump-room the ladies, from time to time, withdraw to a female coffee-house, and from thence return to their lodgings to breakfast. The gentlemen withdraw to their coffee-houses, to read the papers, or converse on the news of the day, with a freedom and ease not to be found in the metropolis.

The rest of the day would be filled with concerts, undemanding lectures, walks and excursions, a further session at the Pump Room and tea at the assembly rooms, followed in the evening by balls, plays and visits. Bath was essentially a social playground for the nobility and gentry, a place to parade one's clothes, wit and gentility – and perhaps one's daughters, in the hope of catching the attention of eligible bachelors. To sip the waters fitted into the social scheme of things better than to bathe, although those with genuine medical problems continued to do so. Even the poor were able to benefit, largely thanks to the work of Dr William Oliver, who founded the Bath General Hospital for – in the words of R.A.L. Smith – 'poor persons who needed the healing waters but could not afford the luxury of being invalids'. Oliver's reward was to come in the form of immortality as the inventor of the Bath Oliver biscuit.

The Bath described by Jane Austen at the dawn of the nineteenth century was a jewel of Georgian architecture but socially a shadow of its former self. All sorts of riff-raff were now turning up, to the extent that the communal amusements previously presided over by Beau Nash were no longer fit for the discerning, who were reduced to organizing their social lives in private. Bath became less of a resort, more a place of retirement, while the fashionable patronized the newer spas such as Cheltenham and Leamington or mingled with European aristocrats at Bad Homburg, Baden-Baden or Aix-les-Bains. Furthermore, sea air and sea-water baths were now being recommended – some daredevils even tried sea bathing – and Brighton, Bournemouth and Boulogne supplanted Bath in royal and then general favour.

10
Enlightenment Strikes the Victorians

Sad to relate, the period known variously as the Age of Enlightenment, of Reason and of Elegance – the age of Voltaire and Mozart, Dean Swift and Thomas Paine, the age in which shibboleths of every kind were swept away by sweet reason – brought little sweetness on the balneological front. While technical advances were proving that there was usually a way, for the most part there simply wasn't the will. Bath and other fashionable European health resorts apart, attitudes to bathing were as negative in the eighteenth century as they had been in the seventeenth. William Thackeray could have been referring to either when he wrote later, in *Pendennis*, 'Gentlemen, there can be but little doubt that your ancestors were the Great Unwashed.' There are reports – disappointing to a patriot – of Englishmen gleefully shaking the bugs out of their wigs in public, and even pitting their lice against each other's in races. It seems unlikely that these included swimming events. As ever, however, there were honourable exceptions, and it is on these that we shall concentrate.

When Laurence Sterne began *A Sentimental Journey Through France and Italy* (1768) with the memorable words, '"They order," said I, "this matter better in France,"' he could easily have been referring to baths. For a century or more, at least at the palatial end of the market, the French had been leading the field. Although Louis XIV is regularly referred to as a once-a-year bather, this is almost certainly a libel. We know, for example, that in the late 1670s alone no fewer than six marble baths were installed in his bathing suite at Versailles. It seems unlikely that the Sun King would have gone to such lengths if he had no interest in bathing. Furthermore, he went on to install a vast octagonal bath of pink marble, six feet in width, the use of which involved submersible cushions and drapery, canopies and curtains. Perhaps it was this bath that he used but once a year. Meanwhile it is recorded that, in all, Versailles had 100 bathrooms as well as over 250 *chaises percées*, or close stools – hardly the arrangements of one whose intentions were not serious. We are told also that Louis washed himself 'with spirit', meaning presumably either that when not actually in the tub he used something like eau-de-cologne – widely preferred to soap, which was thought to coarsen the skin – or that he sang while he bathed.

Over his son Louis XV hangs a question mark. All we know for certain is that he gave away the great octagonal bath – to his mistress Madame de Pompadour – and that it took 22 men to move it. The Pompadour's bathroom was noted for the inclusion of 'English paper' – probably a reference to wallpaper – among its advantages. (The French, incidentally, called the water closet a *lieu à l'anglaise*, meaning 'English place', which was either an insult or suggests that the English were doing something right. There never has been a generally acceptable word for it in English, but from the French *lieu* came the popular nickname of loo – now widely used in lieu, as it were, of a genteel term.) The normal rule in French palace bathrooms of the eighteenth century was to have two baths, so that one could wash in one and rinse off in the other. They would be mounted next to a wall, with hot water piped through from a boiler on the other side. The baths would have canopies and curtains to trap the beneficial steam. Marie Antoinette was in the habit of using only one of her baths, *but used it every day*.

It was not just the Ancien Régime who appreciated luxury. The Princess Borghese, better known as Napoleon's sister Pauline, had a penchant for bathing in milk. Unlike Nero's wife Poppaea, however, she was an easy-going girl who never lost sight of her proletarian roots. She never insisted on asses' milk – any milk would do for her. (As Louis Pasteur was not born till 1822, it didn't even need to be pasteurized.) Nor did she mind who saw her, as it were, *au lait*. She would be lifted in and out by her black man-servant, and while soaking in her milky bath would grant audiences to guests of either sex.

In Britain, innovators such as Pepys's friend Povey were rare. Until the problems of water supply began to be over-come in the second half of the eighteenth century, the most noteworthy achievements were to be found in country mansions. In 1697 Celia Fiennes visited Chatsworth, in Derbyshire, while the house was in the course of being enlarged by the First Duke of Devonshire, and where a convenient supply of water from the moors above the house was being put to good use. Not only had ten water closets been installed: 'There is a fine grotto,' she wrote in her journal, 'within this is a bathing room, the walls all with blue and white marble, the pavement mix'd one stone white, another black, another of the red rance marble; the bath is one entire marble all white finely veined with blue and is made smooth . . . it was as deep as one's middle on the outside, and you went down steps into the bath big enough for two people; at the upper end are two cocks to let in, one hot the other cold, water to attemper it as per-sons please . . .' The Duke appears to have had everything sorted.

At Carshalton in Surrey, Sir John Fellowes went one better. In 1720 he built a fine castellated water-tower over a stream, and used an engine powered by a mill-wheel to pump water up into a lead cistern. Thus water was supplied both to the house and to the boiler room and the bathing room, with its Dutch tiles and marble floor, at the foot of the tower. Presumably he could have had bathrooms with running water all over the house, but perhaps he liked bathing to the sound of the mill-race.

The eighteenth century, however, saw little progress on the plumbing front, and such ventures were the exception rather than the rule. A more usual arrangement was for baths to be filled, albeit on an irregular basis, from rainwater cisterns. In long hot summers, how the committed bather must have yearned for the weather to break. Generally, the motivation to bathe was pretty weak, while in any case the wealthy had plenty of servants to carry water about. Many a bather felt too, as Oscar Wilde did even a century later, that if he wanted hot water he preferred to ring for it.

Meanwhile the medical profession in general and Dr Oliver (he of the biscuit) in particular had been advocating cold bathing. Cold plunge baths became a regular feature of the country house, and at Claremont, in Surrey, Lord Clive had one in his basement. More often it would be in the open air and in the cool shade of trees, as at Rousham in Oxfordshire, in a grotto, as at Stourhead in Wiltshire, or in an ornamental bath-house somewhere in the grounds.

In London, where households had depended on private wells, collecting rainwater or deliveries by watermen, a growing band of private water companies were supplying water piped under the streets through wooden mains. Mostly it came down from Hertfordshire and Hampstead, powered by gravity, but in the 1760s the New River Company began using a steam pump. The problem, apart from the lack of a drainage system, was that the pressure required to supply water to upper floors was too much for the joints of the wooden pipes, and the companies could therefore only supply it at ground level. Iron pipes had been regarded as prohibitively expensive for normal purposes, but in 1817, in order to prevent further damage to the infrastructure through leakage, they were made compulsory. With that, upper floors could be supplied, and demand for water grew rapidly as bathrooms and WCs proliferated. In fact, demand outstripped supply, and the companies were forced to charge more for supplying upper floors, which temporarily put a brake on the bathroom boom.

Even where the technology was available – and in numerous streets and districts it was not – and money no object, the bathroom was far from being an overnight sensation. In 1837, on Queen Victoria's accession, there was no bathroom in Buckingham Palace, and for the time being she made do with a piped supply of hot water to a portable bath in her bedroom. (In later years at Osborne she would bathe in a style befitting the Empress of India, her bath having brass taps of monumental size.) Nor did US Presidents have the use of a bathroom in the White House until 1851 – from which we may deduce that President Millard Fillmore, now remembered chiefly for his failure to reconcile North and South and thus to avert civil war, had at least the satisfaction of one solid achievement. (Just a decade earlier, according to the *News of the World*, the bathtub had been denounced as 'an epicurean innovation from England, designed to corrupt the democratic simplicity of the Republic'. There is no pleasing some people.)

In large houses there was at least scope for converting spare rooms into bathrooms. By the 1870s the typical English country house had one for every three or four bedrooms. Not everyone saw the need, however, and by the time of Charles Darwin's death in 1882 his theory of evolution had not stretched to installing even primordial bathing facilities at Down House. His granddaughter Gwen Raverat would later write, recalling idyllic childhood holidays there in the 1890s, 'There was no bathroom at Down, nor any hot water, except in the kitchen, but there were plenty of housemaids to run about with big brown-painted bath-cans.'

When designing new houses, architects and builders still thought twice about incorporating bathrooms. By the middle of the nineteenth century most upmarket houses included them, but the average suburban one did not. The model cottage designed by Prince Albert for the Great Exhibition of 1851 had a WC but no bathroom. By the end of the century, every newly built suburban villa and all but the smallest London houses had one. For many, therefore, the nineteenth-century bathing experience remained a downstairs one, often involving the wheeling or dragging of a tin bath to the stove and filling it by hand. At least, however, there was a range of portable baths from which to choose.

At the bottom of the range was the sponge bath. This was a round, shallow bath with splayed sides in which you sat or knelt and, by dint of much sponging and doubtless splashing, could just about manage to have a thorough wash with a minimum of water. Not very restful, and not for the arthritic. The oval hip bath, with its raised back, was a slightly better bet, but was so small that only the middle part of the body was submerged, while one's upper half protruded and one's legs dangled. The experience would have dismayed a Roman, but these baths were at least a practical solution where water or space was scarce; likewise the folding bath. More satisfactory was the full bath, or 'ordinary lounge bath', roughly the shape of a modern bath, sometimes with a high back, in which, if enough water was available, you could have a proper soak. The arrival of the gas geyser in 1868 made the full bath – and bigger baths in general – a much more feasible proposition. Now at last the ordinary householder could aspire to an almost Minoan level of luxury.

All these baths were made of copper, zinc or sheet metal coated with paint or a primitive enamel. The latter could be a problem, as Mr Pooter discovered in the Grossmiths' *Diary of a Nobody*. He painted his bath red and, having run from his geyser 'a bath as hot as I could bear it' in order to combat a chill, found that the paint dissolved . . .

Two other Victorian bath types could be mistaken for

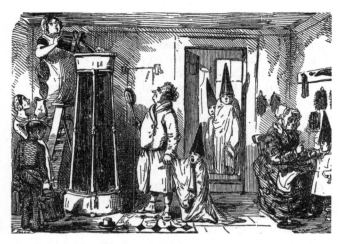

A high-spirited family visit to the shower-bath, drawn by John Leech, 1861.

instruments of torture. The metal slipper bath, or *sabot* in French, was so called because it was shaped like a boot, and the bather was enclosed except for the head and shoulders. This must have prolonged the warmth of the water and produced a sense of wellbeing – unless or until, like the French revolutionary leader Jean Marat, you received a visit from a knife-wielding assassin. There were also various forms of box-like vapour or hot-air bath, in which the bather was not only trapped by the neck but locked in from outside and hazardously heated from inside by a kettle or spirit lamp. These contraptions apparently relieved numerous ailments – while probably inducing acute paranoia.

A happier invention was the shower-bath. This consisted of a hip or sponge bath surmounted by a tank on stilts from which water rained down – but only as long as you kept it filled, either with buckets or a hand pump. The inconvenience (and possible health hazard) of getting water on one's hair was neatly averted by the use of a conical oil-skin shower-cap. In 1849 a friend of the novelist Charlotte Brontë sent her one of these contraptions as a present, and one hopes it was the de luxe model with the hand pump. It is pleasant to imagine the author of *Jane Eyre* pumping away in her shower-cap while wrestling with the plotting problems of *Shirley* or *Villette*.

A civilized and labour-saving Parisian custom among those with the means to pay but apartments too small for a permanent bath was to hire one – hot water included. Transported from the bathing establishment on a cart, the bath would be brought upstairs to your room at the appointed time and removed again a couple of hours later. This practice continued well into the twentieth century.

In Britain, as elsewhere, only the prosperous had access to hot water in the mid-nineteenth century. The poor had always been strangers to the bath, but what used to be a deprivation was now contributing to a disaster. In over-crowded cities with unhygienic living conditions, out-breaks of typhoid, cholera and smallpox were claiming thousands of lives. One of the great achievements of the Victorians was to tackle the issue of public health. In London a new sewerage system was built in 1865, the brainchild of Sir Joseph Bazalgette, Chief Engineer to the Board of Works, and within five years the ravages of cholera had almost ceased. The near death from typhoid of the Prince of Wales in 1871 led to a campaign to improve plumbing standards and eradicate once and for all the insanitary conditions on which disease thrived. This was achieved partly by legislation and partly by the successful, if sanctimonious, equation of cleanliness with respectability.

Parliament had already passed a series of Public Health Acts, among the earliest of which was the Baths and Wash-Houses Act of 1846. This authorized local councils to fund the erection of public baths and wash-houses out of the rates. The grandiose ecclesiastical style of these new institutions reflected the reverence which cleanliness was now accorded. Soon it was possible for people of every class and income bracket to enjoy a cheap if probably rather dismal bath. Dismal or not, for a time the weekly bath became something of a national institution. At the end of the week's work on Saturday afternoons you could wander down to the baths after lunch, wash off the grime and, on emerging, change into clean clothes. As long as you belonged to the 'labouring classes', you could normally have a cold bath for a penny and a warm shower or vapour bath for tuppence. Others paid two or three times as much. Doubtless, arguments arose about the social status of potential bathers, and one wonders how they were settled. For borderline cases, this enlightened system must often have given rise to an agonizing choice between the conflicting demands of snobbishness and economy.

One establishment in Marylebone, London, offered 107 individual baths, as well as vapour baths, showers and two swimming pools. There was an enthusiastic market for swimming, even if segregation of the sexes meant that pleasure stopped some way short of abandon, and pools soon became a routine and popular adjunct to the otherwise utilitarian wash-house. Thus, from about 1880, evolved the municipal swimming pool, which would continue to have a place in British urban life long after the need for public wash-houses had passed.

By this time sea bathing was firmly established as one of the joys of summer, the seaside holiday now made possible for the masses by the growth of the railway network. Once again it was the medical profession which had set the ball rolling, when royalty and fashion descended on Brighton and Weymouth in order, at first, to drink sea water, albeit 'mixed with port wine, milk or beef tea to make it more palatable'. To this penance was added the dubious privilege

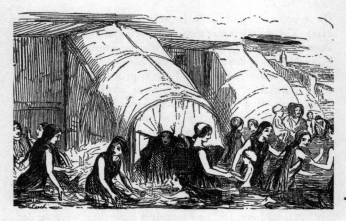

Girls bathing from machines fitted with the 'modesty hood', drawn by John Leech, 1861.

of being lowered into tanks of sea water by a hired 'dipper' – but at least this must have been better than taking the stuff internally.

Bathing in the sea itself was made possible for the squeamish by the use of the bathing machine, a glorified horse-drawn cart which was wheeled into the water and turned around, so that bathers could lower themselves into the waves from its rear. Its glory lay in the 'modesty hood', a huge awning which screened the bathers from the eyes and telescopes of landlubbers. (This Margate invention was not used everywhere, which led to Brighton, for example, gaining a somewhat louche reputation.) Mixed bathing was strictly prohibited everywhere for most of the Victorian age – beaches being divided into separate areas and fines imposed on transgressors and those who came too close in boats – and nude bathing was out of the question. Ladies were at first so heavily swathed that swimming would have been difficult even if it had not still been the custom to be 'dipped' by the hired help; men, for fear of inflaming the women, had to wear costumes which covered their chests.

By the 1870s, things had loosened up a bit, but not enough for the Reverend Francis Kilvert, who in 1873 nearly got into hot water at Seaton, in Dorset. The previous year, at the more informal Weston-super-Mare, Kilvert had enjoyed 'a delicious feeling of freedom in stripping in the open air and running naked down to the sea'. At Seaton he found that things were ordered differently, as he recorded in his diary:

While Dora was sitting on the beach I had a bathe. A boy brought me to the machine door two towels as I thought, but when I came out of the water and began to use them I found that one of the rags he had given me was a pair of very short red and white striped drawers to cover my nakedness. Unaccustomed to such things and customs I had in my ignorance bathed naked and set at nought the conventionalities of the place and scandalized the beach.

As the old century drew to a close, the bathing machines were being replaced by gaudy tents, and segregation was less rigorously enforced; as the new one dawned, a few permissive places such as Bexhill-on-Sea even took a deep breath and gave the go-ahead to 'promiscuous' or mixed bathing.

11
The Bath Rampant

'The bathroom is a perfect boon to those who like washing.'

So the *Builder* magazine pronounced in 1904, inscrutably bestowing approval while also withholding it. This masterly piece of equivocation from the voice of the British building trade, at once categorical and doubtful, reflects the position of the bath at the turn of the century. It was here to stay, and on the verge of being rampant, but its universal presence was still a long way off.

Hotels had for some time been making the running towards baths for all, not least in the USA. The massive Mount Vernon Hotel in Cape May, New Jersey, built in 1853, had been the first to boast of a bath with hot and cold water in every bedroom. The next step forward was taken in London. After the luxurious new Savoy Hotel (built 1884–9) had made a splash by advertising no fewer than 67 bathrooms, the Carlton (1891–9) became the first hotel to provide every bedroom with a bathroom of its own. It was in the USA, however, that this luxury was made generally affordable, the new Statler Hotel in Buffalo proving an instant hit in 1908 with its motto, 'A Room and a Bath for a Dollar and a Half'.

Meanwhile, on both sides of the Atlantic, many houses still had no bathroom, and public baths were far from sufficient to cater for everyone. 'Even in 1908 in London,' notes Lawrence Wright in *Clean and Decent*, 'there was only one municipal tub for about 2,000 inhabitants. The Cheyenne Indians, the Hawaiians, the Baganda of East Africa and the Chiriguano of the South American Chaco were still well ahead of the Londoner in the matter of daily bathing.'

If, numerically, the rampancy of the bath was still to

come, aesthetically its heyday had begun. The first great watershed had been the Victorian invention of the afore-mentioned gas geyser. Consisting of a tube of water coiling or zigzagging its way past a row of gas burners, the geyser has had a distinguished career, especially once having become more user-friendly with the introduction of the pilot light. It remains a very practical way of heating exactly the required amount of water, and doing it on the spot, with no wasteful loss of heat along yards of pipe.

In its explosive early days the geyser had competition from the no less intimidating gas bath. Here gas burners were applied directly to the underside of the bath, which became, in effect, a giant saucepan. The risks were obvious. Ewart's classic model, the 'General Gordon' (see cover illustration) – with its ornate towel-warmer as an exquisite little annexe – was launched in 1882, the year of the Mahdi's revolt in the Sudan. Three years later under the burning African sun, the General would have felt no need for the bath named after him, but if news of this terror machine had been allowed to spread among the Mahdi's followers, one wonders whether Khartoum would ever have been seriously threatened. (For those with a taste for danger, there was also a cheaper, portable gas water heater which could be connected to a gas light bracket, and which you actually had in the water with you. It scarcely bears thinking about, and it is astonishing to learn that it was still around in the 1920s.)

With supplies of hot water available from the geyser, the days of the portable bath were numbered. Instead of lurk-ing in a corner of the bedroom, the bath would now be in permanent situ; and thus was the bathroom proper born, whether purpose-built, as was increasingly the case, or con-verted from another use. Now there was nothing to stop baths getting bigger and heavier, and the designers and sani-tary engineers, already responsible for an explosion of inno-vation in the WC, eagerly turned their attention to the bath.

The first step was to cast decorative supports. These were often in the form of clawed feet or classical plinths, while the Bolding company produced a bath supported, more appropriately, by dolphins. Shanks too favoured piscine motifs, offering their 'Fin de Siècle' cast-iron bath with a raised pattern of plunging dolphins. (If you didn't want fish, you could have bunches of grapes.) The disadvantage of the cast-iron bath with its japanned finish (usually fake wood or marble) was that it needed frequent repainting. The ceramic bath was longer lasting and therefore preferable, for those who could afford it.

If you really wanted to impress your guests, you had the bath encased in mahogany or oak, with a hooded shower cabinet at the end. In this case you would have a veritable battery of taps to operate. Apart from the hot and cold taps, there would be one to fill the bath, one for a gentle shower, one for a 'douche' (a virtual waterfall from the middle of the shower rose), one for a 'spray' or 'needle bath' (horizontal sprinklers from all sides, along the lines of a car-wash), and another to empty the bath. All being well, you could feel not just in control, but like the Chief Engineer on a steamship.

At the luxurious end of the market, Victorian and Edwardian designers indulged their clients' or their own more exuberant fancies. After all, why bother with marbling effects, as the sanitary ware manufacturers did, if you could use marble? At Cardiff Castle, William Burges designed a bathroom for Lord Bute that was all marble and mahogany. His Lordship's marble Roman bath was decorated in metal with denizens of the deep, including a starfish around the plughole. At Port Lympne, in Kent, Philip Sassoon had an array of extravagant bathrooms, his own having a Roman bath of red marble, as well as a Roman swimming pool. Meanwhile, at the prosaic-sounding address of 8 Addison Road, London W.14, Sir Ernest Debenham's Oriental dream house was taking shape;

among its exotic wonders was a bathroom fitted throughout with tilework by William de Morgan depicting
mythical beasts – a Persian phantasmagoria swathing a
'Tubular, Spray, Shower and Wave Bath' by Shanks.

It has been said that England entered the twentieth century looking backwards. There was indeed a nostalgic
romanticism about the Arts and Crafts-influenced country
house architecture of Lutyens and others which often led
to modern innovations such as garages being heavily dis-
guised. There was no escaping the new bathroom technology, however – whatever William Morris would have said
about it. The clients wanted it, and in any case it was hid-
den from view. So in the bathroom, as Mark Girouard puts
it, 'country-house architects tended to let themselves go,
and indulge in untraditional and often expensive fantasies
in glass, marble, metal and mosaic' – the hard surfaces
which suited the bathroom also happening to lend themselves to Art Deco design. Sir James Miller, at Manderston,
must have felt that he had transcended architectural fashion
as he he gazed up at his groined vault of marble – from his
silver-plated tub. Lutyens himself designed eight bathrooms for Gledstone Hall, in Yorkshire, and fourteen for
Middleton Park, in Oxfordshire. As early as 1905, for Lady
Wimborne, he even produced drawings of a bathroom containing a sunken bath in an alcove shaped like a seashell. It
seems, however, that Her Ladyship never was to arise like
Venus – or Britannia – from her ocean scallop. Did
Lutyens, perhaps, who was only 36, fail to conceal a snig-
ger, so that she lost her nerve – and he the job ?

There was nothing bashful about Stephen Courtauld,
who in the 1930s built his Art Deco mansion, Courtauld
House, at Eltham – now a South London suburb – on the
site of the former royal palace and incorporating its sole
survival, the Great Hall. His wife Virginia had a bathroom
which was and still is the highlight of any tour, with its
onyx bath, gold-plated fittings and a recess tiled in gold

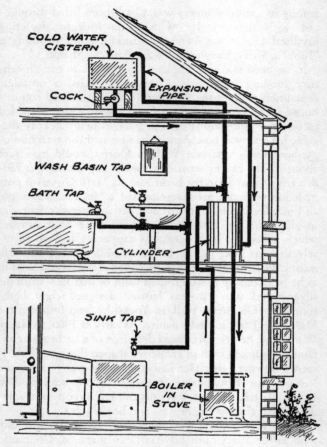

COLD WATER CISTERN

EXPANSION PIPE.

COCK

WASH BASIN TAP

BATH TAP

CYLINDER

SINK TAP.

BOILER IN STOVE

Children will ask questions like 'How do we get hot water?' This is one answer.

mosaic which used to house a marble statue of Psyche. Unfortunately Stephen Courtauld felt the need to be able to address the entire household at any time; he therefore installed a tannoy system with speakers in every room – which must have rather defeated the object of his wife's bathroom. In fact they stayed there only six years before leaving for Southern Rhodesia.

Pride of place for twentieth-century ostentation should perhaps go to a Mrs Cromwell, an American described by the *Daily Mail* in 1938 as 'reputed to be the world's richest woman', whose Honolulu home, according to the paper, had excellent facilities: 'Around the base of the walls in Mrs Cromwell's bathroom are slabs of white marble two feet square, each inlaid with jade and semi-precious marbles forming bright flowers and other designs.'

Back in the real world, another watershed period was that following the First World War. Except where the geyser was still appropriate – for example in rented accommodation – hot water was already being supplied by the system which remains the norm today, incorporating a boiler at ground level and a hot-water cylinder above, and was being used more liberally than ever. In this one sense at least, Britain was indeed becoming a land fit for heroes to live in. Before the war, Elder Duncan had written: 'Educated people look upon their baths as an enjoyable pleasure, and not, like many of our forefathers, as a necessary but troublesome item of cleanliness to be undertaken with fear and trembling and extraordinary preparations and precautions.' Now that almost every new home came equipped with a bathroom, that change in attitude was no longer confined to the educated classes. For the miner, meanwhile, sitting in his tin bath in the kitchen after a hard day at the coal face, just as his father had done, such talk of new homes and changing attitudes would have raised at best a rueful smile. For many people nothing was changing.

In the brave new world that followed the Second World War the government set about improving living conditions in older houses. One of the provisions of the 1949 Housing

Act was that an owner who wished to install a bathroom could claim a grant of £100. Such measures, together with growing prosperity over the next few decades, have so reduced the pockets of resistance to the spread of the bath that in Britain it really does seem to be virtually universal. Even the smallest council flat now has its own bathroom, which has come to be regarded as a basic human right.

In some places, one must in fairness state, the shower has replaced the bath. There are even those who will argue for the superiority of the shower, which admittedly is more economical, quicker to use, easier to share and certainly more hygienic, but otherwise has nothing to recommend it. Its advantages are obvious and irrelevant. Apart from anything else, you can read in the bath, or fall asleep. The first is virtually impossible in a shower; the second, positively dangerous. However, there is no sense in getting involved in this negative argument.

If the price of the bath's near universality used to be a depressingly functional uniformity – Victorians and Edwardians had a far greater choice of designs than was available in the 1950s – recent years have seen a welcome improvement. Ceramic, acrylic and steel baths are available in a wide range of elegant styles, some of which show subtle influences of an earlier period; while those who respond to the monumental solidity of Tower Bridge or the Great Western Railway can create a bathing ambience that is heavily Victorian.

Bathroom technology has also reached a level of sophistication that even a Roman would envy. While regretting the demise of the strigil and the ever reliable hypocaust, he or she would doubtless admire the quietly flushing loo, the heated towel rail, the mixer tap and the wonders of electricity, from the dimmer switch and the electric rasor to, above all, the instant availability of hot water, its temperature thermostatically controlled, in bath, shower, jacuzzi or whirlpool at the touch of a button.

Having admired all these mod cons, however, the Roman would very likely grow restless after observing how the bathroom is used, and eventually say, 'But where's the fun?' For while the possibilities of private bathing are now surely greater than they have ever been, for those who have the means, there is no likelihood that public baths or communal bathing will ever again occupy a central position in daily life. In Roman times the baths were a communal institution with an unhurried routine – a kind of reviving, hygienic, sociable, often rather immoral but immensely enjoyable club that everyone could join. There are clubs today, of course, but the modern health club is used in a different way. The people who can afford it tend to be too busy to use it except for short, frenetic visits squeezed into hectic schedules; and it is too narrowly focused on the needs of the individual, as well as being too 'exclusive' to bear comparison. As for the swimming pool, it would certainly be entertaining to see a Roman's reaction to the wave machine and the flume (which even for the Romans would have been taxing to build in stone), but otherwise it is an overtly sport-based and utilitarian development of what for the Romans was just one feature among many.

Meanwhile there are establishments offering saunas and massage, and it seems appropriate that once again such places have acquired the louche reputation previously enjoyed by the hothouse, bagnio or stew. In many cases this is almost certainly unfair, while others, one is given to understand, do indeed offer a wide range of services not always available elsewhere.

Doubtless there are those who try to use the health club or the swimming pool – surely not the massage parlour – for hygienic, fitness and social purposes, and perhaps even emerge morally as well as physically refreshed; none of these places, however, will ever attract such a broad cross section of society, day in, day out, and play such a central role in the daily life of society as did the Greek and Roman baths. Apart from anything else, while swimming may be communal, bathing proper, which involves removal of the clothes and a relaxed attitude to nudity, surely never will be again. Modesty has seen to that. Truth to tell, she has a great deal to answer for.

12
The Bath in Art

The bathtub does not play a prominent role in the history of art. Until the nineteenth century, the subject was regarded as being too mundane and private for the serious artist. A bathing occasion which had historical significance was a different matter, and the Old Testament story of David and Bathsheba hinges on just such an event. Bathsheba, the wife of Uriah the Hittite, was observed bathing by King David from the roof of his palace. Deeply smitten, he wanted her for himself, and his integrity was put to the test. It failed, and in order to get her husband out of the way he arranged for Uriah to lead their army into battle and be left without support. The plan worked: Uriah was killed, David and Bathsheba were married, and although God punished David by having their first child die, Bathsheba later gave birth to Solomon, beginning a line that ended with Joseph, the husband of the Virgin Mary. Thus the charming sight of Bathsheba bathing led indirectly to Bethlehem and the Christian faith – although if God had been just that little bit angrier, one imagines that he might well have called the whole Messiah project off, or at least used a different family.

This fateful bath has been depicted many times, not always as one would have wished. In medieval miniatures and at least one seventeenth-century Flemish painting Bathsheba is shown merely drying herself after washing at a fountain. Earlier this century, however, Marc Chagall struck a blow for the bath. His charming etching 'David and Bathsheba' shows her standing thigh-deep in what looks like a serious tub, watched from above by David, who leans precariously from his battlements.

The most celebrated bathtub painting depicts a more

recent and more melodramatic bathing occasion. The eighteenth-century French doctor turned journalist turned revolutionary leader Jean Marat was soaking – and working – in his tub one day when he received a visitor. This, unluckily for him, was the young Charlotte Corday, whose lover had been among those Marat had sent to the guillotine, and who had come to settle up. Producing a knife from her basket, she stabbed him through the heart. In Jacques David's famous painting, 'The Dead Marat', he is shown in a romantic pose, slumped against the side of the tub with one arm dangling pathetically, his quill still clutched in his hand. In fact we know that Marat, who spent much of his time in the bath, which he used as an office, on account of a painful skin disease, favoured a slipper bath. Thus the picture reproduced here is historically more accurate than David's painting. The latter, in his revolutionary zeal, probably felt that a bath which made the martyred Marat look like a 1950s racing driver was insufficiently heroic and picturesque.

Hothouse bathing figured, as we have seen, in the work of Albrecht Dürer, who drew men and women steaming away in the vapour baths of fifteenth-century Nuremberg in a woodcut and a pen-and-ink drawing respectively; it was also treated by Jean Ingres in his 'Turkish Bath' of 1859.

When it comes to realism in bathing art, there is only one champion: Edgar Degas. His predilection for painting ordinary, often weary-looking women performing their ablutions is one of the traits which set him apart from his Impressionist colleagues. It was largely a desire to escape such scenes, no doubt, that led Monet, Pissarro and others to take their easels out into the fields. What the models who posed for Degas would have said about his requirements is anybody's guess. Often the wretched girl would have to squat, kneel or try to wash her hair in a sponge bath so pitifully shallow that it looks more like a dustbin

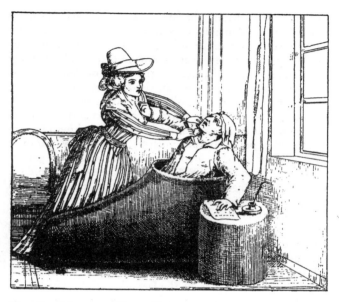

How Jean Marat actually got his come-uppance.

lid. Even when the girls were allowed to pose in the artist's own bath, life was not much easier: he tended to want to paint them getting in or out rather than actually bathing, and this would often involve standing on one leg in the bath or, bent double, with one leg in and the other on the floor. Painful cramps must have been an occupational hazard. One hopes, at least, that Degas had the decency to keep the bath water tolerably warm.

No such problems presumably beset the models who posed for his contemporary, Sir Lawrence Alma-Tadema. Quite apart from the fact that he tended to use his nearest and dearest as models, his bathing scenes could hardly be more different from those of Degas, either in subject matter or in execution. Riding the late Victorian vogue for classical extravaganzas, Alma-Tadema depicted thinly draped and sometimes naked women in languid, graceful poses amid the marble splendours of the great Roman thermae. Everything is so graceful, if not genteel, at the Baths of Alma-Tadema that one would scarcely be surprised to see a notice on the wall, hanging from a wholly authentic peg, saying 'No squatting'. To his credit, when it comes to authenticity of historical and architectural detail, the painstaking research and technical perfectionism which went into his vast canvases leave nothing to be desired. He was also a brilliant painter of stone: unkind critics have suggested that there is more life in his marbles than in his figures. However, even if he used the classical Roman setting chiefly to provide a cloak of respectability and a means of getting nude figures past the moral watchdogs of the Royal Academy, the world would be a poorer place without at least a few magnificent visions such as 'The Baths of Caracalla'.

Huge effects being beyond the scope of the theatre, such populist art was in a sense the late Victorian equivalent of cinema. Alma-Tadema certainly painted on an epic scale, just as the Romans bathed, and if artistically he was no Eisenstein, he could probably be regarded as the Cecil B. deMille of his age.

When the cinema did arrive, to become the most popular art form of the masses, it was chariot races that they mostly got; but the bath has nonetheless played an honourable role – if generally a comic or glamorous one rather than an epic one. It has frequently been used as a comic 'rite of passage' symbol to mark an earthy character's entry into polite society or indeed marriage. In the 1964 film *My Fair Lady*, Audrey Hepburn as Eliza Dolittle is forcibly bathed on being received into the Higgins household, while Lee Marvin as the hard-living Ben is likewise encouraged to make himself more wholesome when about to marry Maria (Jean Seberg) in the 1969 *Paint Your Wagon*. Both these characters betray the fact that they are strangers to the bath. Children, too, are routinely pushed into baths, protesting noisily, when their urchin days are over.

In political and crime thrillers, corpses turn up in baths with monotonous regularity. There is something particularly gruesome about violent death in a place which gives such a sense of privacy and security. In some cases, however, the body is just dumped in the bath, the deed having been done elsewhere. In the case of a bloody corpse this is clearly practical – it saves no end of mess. It may seem odd that anyone who has just stabbed or bludgeoned someone to death should be concerned about the decor, but that is the kind of civilization we live in. Never mind the victim – is the carpet all right?

One of the more original uses of a bathing ambience for cinematic violence occurs in the 1983 thriller *Gorky Park*. Having solved the murders, the William Hurt character goes to a luxury Moscow bath-house for a confrontation with the menacing KGB bigwig played by Ian Bannen, and there is a satisfyingly gory denouement. The scene was shot in the real-life Sandunovsky Baths, a much-loved institution where for a hundred years Muscovites have gone for a sauna and perhaps a bit of flagellation with a birch, followed by a cold plunge and a vodka. It was in the Sandunovsky pool, incidentally, that Sergei Eisenstein, using model ships, had filmed parts of *Battleship Potemkin*.

The bath has also provided some of Hollywood's brighter and more glamorous moments. Betty Grable, favourite GI pin-up of the Second World War, played one particular bathing scene in which she proved to be not just alluring but inspirational. In the 1943 musical *Sweet Rosie O'Grady*, about an Irish-American singing star, there is a scene in which Grable rehearses a new song while relaxing in a bubble bath. She not only sings it perfectly first time but does it without the slightest impairment of her make-up or hair-do. Although modestly swathed in bubbles throughout, she caused a sensation and possibly shortened the war. In no time at all Montgomery's Eighth Army was sweeping westwards from El Alamein, while the British and American forces under Eisenhower thrust eastwards from Casablanca, and by the end of May Rommel's *Wehrmacht* had been flushed out of Africa. The Germans had decisively lost the initiative and were never to regain it.

An unusual 'reverse drag' bathing scene occurs in Billy Wilder's 1959 comedy *Some Like It Hot*. Tony Curtis, known to all but Jack Lemmon as Josephine, the saxophonist in the all-girl jazz band for which Sugar (Marilyn Monroe) sings, has just posed as a sensitive millionaire on the Miami beach and aroused Sugar's interest. When she races back to the hotel to report her news to Josephine, Curtis has to get there even faster . . . 'Josephine' is discovered submerged in bubbles, and only when Sugar exits does Tony Curtis emerge, still wearing the naval blazer and slacks of the yacht-owning 'millionaire' – having almost been caught wearing men's clothes.

Monroe herself, of course, had her moments in the bath, including the odd careless one. A highlight of *The Seven Year Itch* (1955), also directed by Wilder, is the charming scene in which, a victim once again, she gets her toe very sweetly stuck in the tap and has to be rescued by Victor Moore.

The director Billy Wilder, incidentally, was responsible for what must be a rare telegram on a bathing theme. While filming in Paris, he was instructed by his wife to bring back with him a bidet – this French device having taken her fancy during a previous visit there together. With shooting running late, and having no time to carry out this commission, Wilder cabled home: 'REGRET BIDET UNOBTAINABLE STOP SUGGEST HANDSTAND IN SHOWER.'

While the shower does not seem to lend itself to comedy, it can claim to have provided one of the most sensational moments in cinematic history. Janet Leigh, the wife of

Tony Curtis, played a character on the run with stolen loot in Alfred Hitchcock's 1960 thriller *Psycho*. Prudently she turns off the freeway on to the old road, now little used, and pulls in at the Bates Motel. Stepping wearily into a hot shower, she thinks her troubles are over . . . The rest, like her, is history.

It is once again the shower, as it happens, rather than the bath, which figures in the work of the painter who has made the most significant contribution to bathing art in the twentieth century. In the mid-1960s David Hockney became *the* artist of the Californian swimming pool with a series of acrylic paintings including 'The Splash', 'A Bigger Splash' and 'Peter Getting out of Nick's Pool'. In a commentary on these, Hockney was later to observe that whereas the colour of a river is related to the sky it reflects, 'the look of swimming-pool water is controllable . . . and its dancing rhythms reflect not only the sky but, because of its transparency, the depth of the water as well. So I had to use techniques to represent this (later I became more aware of the wetness of the surface).' Hockney brought a similar awareness to bear on another subject that he made his own: the shower. At around the same time he produced another series of acrylics, this time of male nudes in showers, with titles such as 'Boy About to Take a Shower' and 'Man Taking Shower in Beverly Hills'. Here he shows an awareness not only of the watery wetness of the water, but also, most satisfyingly, of the angular tiliness of tiles and the imposing bottomliness of bottoms.

Epilogue
or Running Out

What all the bathing civilizations have in common is a piece of wisdom which goes back many centuries and goes thus: if you suddenly wake up and the water's cold and your fingers have the texture of stewed prunes, it's time to get out. The experience can be annoying, and even – if you also realize that you still haven't done what you came to do, i.e. the soap is still dry – mortifying. Not that it should concern us nowadays. When the bath was at best a weekly privilege, such a lapse would have been a matter for regret, but in these enlightened times tomorrow, as Scarlett says, is another day.

The bath is, after all – you could say above all – a pleasant place to linger, and you are unlikely, asleep or not, to come to any harm. Ah, you may say, try telling that to St Cecilia, Agamemnon, Jean Marat or the Brides in the Bath . . . Certainly one or two people have had unfortunate experiences while bathing – this book would have included a chapter on crimes in the bath had space allowed – but one might as well say, in the light of Abraham Lincoln's fate, that theatre-going must be a hazardous pastime.

I believe, as an Aquarian and a committed bather (albeit an off-peak one, as anyone is liable to be who works at home and shares a bathroom with a wife and three daughters), that the bath has done no harm and quite a lot of good; indeed that it has probably done much to help the human race feel better in itself, and even to civilize it – for it has the power, like music, of soothing savage breasts.